The Practice
of Clinical Psychology
in Great Britain

# The Practice of Clinical Psychology in Great Britain

Edited by

**Andrée Liddell**

*Memorial University of Newfoundland*

JOHN WILEY & SONS

Chichester · New York · Brisbane · Toronto · Singapore

***British Library Cataloguing in Publication Data***

Liddell, Andrée
The practice of clinical psychology in Great Britain.
1. Clinical psychology
I. Title
157′.9 RC467

ISBN 0 471 10288 1

***Library of Congress Cataloging in Publication Data***
Main entry under title:

The Practice of clinical psychology in Great Britain.

Includes index.
1. Clinical psychology—Great Britain. 2. Mental health services—Great Britain. I. Liddell, Andrée.
[DNLM: 1. Psychology, Clinical—Great Britain. WM 105 P895]
RC469.P68 1983 362.2 82-20030

ISBN 0 471 10288 1

Typeset by Inforum Ltd, Portsmouth
Printed in Great Britain by Page Bros (Norwich) Ltd.

# Acknowledgements

Grateful thanks are due to all the contributors who have accepted willingly the most difficult task of describing vast areas in so little space – it turned out to be a fine example of corporate work!

Although Martyn Baker was unable to continue as co-editor after the first year of preparation, he continued to give valuable and valued advice unofici-ally. Unfortunately, May Davidson was unable to write the chapter she had planned to contribute on the development of the profession before her untimely death but she left notes which were incorporated in Chapter 1. Grace Rawlings generously offered many comments and suggestions on the manuscripts of Chapters 1 and 2 and most of her suggestions were gratefully accepted. To both May and Grace, who have been the true pioneers of our profession, too much is due to be adequately expressed here.

The help of both Maureen Lyons and Pat Triggs proved to be invaluable during the last stages of preparation as was the continuous help of Pet Smith who carried out cheerfully and efficiently all the secretarial work involved throughout the editorial work.

Permission was generously granted by the American Psychological Associ-ation to reproduce the three tables which appear in Chapter 15.

A.L.

# *List of Contributors*

Ronald Blackburn, *Department of Psychology, Park Lane Hospital, Magull, Liverpool.*

Peter G. Britton, *Department of Psychiatry, University of Newcastle-upon-Tyne.*

Janet Carr, *Department of Psychiatry, St. George's Hospital Medical School, London.*

Dorothy M. Fielding, *Sub-Department of Clinical Psychology, Liverpool University.*

Sol L. Garfield, *Department of Psychology, Washington University, St Louis, USA.*

Karen Hassel, *Spes klin Psykologi, NPF, Oslo, Norway.*

Lionel R. C. Haward, *Department of Psychology, Surrey University, Guildford.*

Andrée Liddell, *Department of Psychology, Memorial University of Newfoundland, Canada (formerly Clinical Psychology Centre, North East London Polytechnic).*

Nadina Lincoln, *Department of Health Care of the Elderly, Sherwood Hospital, Nottingham.*

Frank M. McPherson, *Tayside Area Clinical Psychology Department, Dundee.*
Edgar Miller, *Department of Clinical Psychology, Addenbrookes Hospital, Cambridge.*

Fraser N. Watts, *MRC Applied Psychology Unit, Cambridge.*

William Yule, *Department of Psychology, Institute of Psychiatry, London.*

# *Contents*

## PART III DEVELOPMENT OF NEW SERVICES



## PART IV CLINICAL PSYCHOLOGISTS IN OTHER COUNTRIES

*Foreword*

# *Clinical Psychology in Britain – Retrospect and Prospect*

*S.J. Rachman*

The timely publication of this book, appearing after the most vigorous growth period of clinical psychology, invites one to consider the path taken by the profession during the past three decades and, inevitably, leads to questions about its future. The expansion which took place in the post-war period, culminating in the recognition of the profession that was implicit in the Trethowan Report, signals a time to take stock. Notwithstanding the serious arguments against establishing a professional framework and semi-medical style for clinical psychology, the Trethowan Report was accepted warmly by a majority of psychologists and marked the coming of age of the profession in this country.

It has been argued that this was a hollow victory because the recommendations, although accepted by the government, were not followed by the provision of the financial support that would have enabled psychologists and others to put the recommendations into action. Never one to turn down an offer of hard cash, I nevertheless feel that the Report was an important achievement for the profession (and its able spokesmen on the Trethowan Committee). Firstly, there was the recognition of the contribution which clinical psychologists can make to health care. Secondly, the Report acknowledged the desirability of fostering the growth of an *independent* profession. Thirdly, the particular contribution which psychologists can and have made to research was recognized, as was the need to expand the scope of psychology to include a wide range of medical problems.

It is true that the recommendations of the Committee, despite their importance, have not spread as widely as one might have hoped. This is a reflection of the relatively small number of psychologists in the country, and also shows a lack of initiative in attempting to persuade, and demonstrate, to related professions the nature and magnitude of their potential contribution.

For the remainder of this introduction, I will attempt to draw attention to specific achievements that were recorded during the first stage of the development of the profession, identify some errors that were made, guess what is likely to happen in the future, and hope what should happen if all goes well. I will include some remarks on the profession as practised in Britain and other countries in Europe, and in North America, as I find myself in the happy position of having worked in three continents (and can, therefore, claim to have just enough experience of other conditions to reflect on the strengths and weaknesses of clinical psychology in this country).

At the outset, it can be said that a great deal of value has been achieved. It is a matter for regret, however, that the knowledge and skills which have been acquired have not been disseminated or used as widely as one might wish. Clinical psychologists have more skills and knowledge than are being used. To take the most obvious example, the provision of a far greater number of psychologists for the care of handicapped people would certainly improve the lives of the many thousands of people who at present receive little or no psychological assistance. The failure to apply the extensive knowledge of the child psychologist to pediatric services is another example of insufficient application.

Leaving aside the insufficient *distribution* of psychological skills, we can concentrate instead on the important achievements recorded so far. Most of my own experience has been in the field of teaching of clinical knowledge and skills, and it is my strong impression that the training provided by the British university courses is excellent, and probably is unmatched in any other country, European or American. British universities have succeeded admirably in pursuing the scientist/practitioner model that was originally endorsed at the Boulder Conference many years ago. While still pursuing that general aim, the British universities diverged from the American ones in not accepting the need for clinical training to be based on a lengthy Ph.D. course. The British teachers also diverged by insisting that clinical teachers should continue to carry out their own clinical work and should be seen to do so. The most serious weakness of North American courses, many of which have individual features which excel those that can be found in any particular British university department, is the large gap between the high quality of university instruction which is provided and the poor and often unsupervised clinical training which the students obtain. The courses are badly unbalanced, and the scientist has squeezed out the practitioner. In many instances, the students are required to make such arrangements as they can for their own clinical training — the university training courses absolve themselves from the responsibility for developing or even selecting clinical training sites, monitoring them, or evaluating what the student has learned. Against this extremely unsatisfactory system, the British insistence on combining the teaching role of academic and clinician has a great deal to recommend it. Although I cannot recall ever having won this particular argument with American colleagues, the excellent quality of British clinical graduates seems to me to justify the local practice of providing a two-year training course, rather than the extraordinarily lengthy courses demanded by American universities.

The competence and confidence with which most graduates leave the British training courses reflect the enormous efforts which most of these students put into their concentrated two-year training course. And when it is argued, as often it is, that these concentrated two-year courses are too tightly packed and that it is unreasonable to expect students to complete research projects while gaining a professional training, one has simply to turn to the record. The overwhelming majority of students who are accepted on these courses complete them successfully and then go on to practise with at least reasonable success, and often with a great deal of success. Judging from Dr Hemsley's as-yet-unpublished report on the research activities of clinical psychologists, disappointingly few graduates undertake research after they have completed their training. However, this finding is consistent with reports from America, in which it is found that more than half of their clinical psychology graduates fail to publish any research after qualifying. It should not be concluded from these figures that the emphasis placed on research training has failed and therefore, is misguided. It may be necessary to provide such experience for the many in order to encourage the few. There is the further argument that a period of carrying out one's own research is an excellent foundation for evaluating the professional literature. Carrying out a research project increases one's sense of realism, among its other benefits.

As far as the provision of services is concerned, this subject is well-covered in the book, and here it is necessary merely to say that there has been a welcome expansion of psychological services during the past six years. This next development, which should be encouraged as a priority, is an expansion beyond the original scope of psychology as a sub-speciality of psychiatric medicine, to include the full range of health services. In the recent past, valuable progress has been made in extending psychological services to handicapped people and the elderly. During the next few years, we shall see a greater provision of psychological care in primary health settings, and even in social service departments.

Against a general background of progress and achievement, what failings and errors can be identified? On the teaching side, we have perhaps been too slow in expanding the horizons and perspectives of our students. It took far too long to make the move from an almost exclusive concern with psychiatric psychology to the wider aspects of health care service. A finger could also be pointed at the inadequacy of our training in basic psychological skills such as interviewing. The great problem with many of these wholly desirable aims, however, is that the knowledge on which one would like to proceed is deficient or equivocal. Another failing of the educational side of the profession can be seen in our lack of success in persuading students to show any enthusiasm for working with populations of handicapped people. These seem always to be the last jobs to be filled, and we have yet to find a way to generate the necessary enthusiasm and motivation; there remains a great need for psychologists to do this invaluable work. Another failing is seen in our inability to persuade more of our graduates to include active research as part of their personal 'job description'. This is not to say that all graduates can or should be capable of carrying out important creative research. Nevertheless, there are few clinical posts in which some research is neither possible nor desirable. One way or another, means should be found to ensure that the university training prepares the clinical psychologist to continue his own research after qualification. This is necessary for the vitality of the subject and the profession.

On the provision of services, the failings mostly have been those of slowness. For too long, we continued passively to accept the role of testers, even when our instruments were being used indiscriminately and without sufficient justification. The era of test-bashing continued for an undue length of time. The effort and thought that went into testing those many thousands of patients could more profitably have been spent providing them with other forms of psychological assistance. Because the testing period extended beyond its sensible scope and lasted far too long, it was wasteful, but as far as I am aware, was not too damaging.

On the research side, the main complaint is that insufficient emphasis is placed on this part of our work, and it can be added that a great deal of the published research seems to be of little importance. This might be an inevitable reflection of the enormous volume of material which is published each month, but in any event, there are days on which the appearance of a new issue is greeted by dismay rather than pleasure.

Relative to the provision of services in other countries, my impression is that British psychologists are doing at least as well as and probably better than most of their colleagues in other countries. To a large extent, this has been made possible by the sensible use of psychologists within the National Health system. With their increasing independence, it is to be hoped that in future the limited resources available to psychologists will be deployed with greater effect than in the past. The district psychological team will be in a far stronger position to determine the priorities and the correct distribution of the limited resources. It is rare to find a comparable set of NHS arrangements in other countries, and as a result, foreign psychological services tend to be even more patchy. In some settings, the services provided in Britain are superlative, but serious shortages remain. The overall quality of the service seems to be high.

Like all of the health care professions, we have to take into account the profound change in attitude towards public expenditure that has taken place during the past few years. We will not be functioning in an ever-expanding world of limitless resources. A short period of retrenchment certainly is to be expected, but my belief is that a return to mildly expansionary policies will then take place as a result of technological changes, which will in turn give rise to economic policies that will usher in a different sort of expansion. It will be necessary to find useful non-productive (in the material sense) employment for an ever increasing number of people. Provision of health and education will, therefore, receive an increasingly large portion of the national budget. Yet these same technological advances will change drastically the way in which psychologists function. To take the most obvious, but by no means the least important change, the great amount of time taken up by the administration and scoring of psychological tests will soon become unnecessary. The face-to-face 'hand administration' of psychological tests will be as anachronistic as computing correlations with a pad and pencil. The introduction of microprocessors, which are easily capable of administering and scoring psychological tests, signals the end of conventional testing as we know it. What then will psychologists do with their new liberty?

The advances in electronic apparatus will enable us to collect and analyse vast amounts of data, on a scale previously unimagined. Rickety old baseline recording, in which patients laboriously scratch the odd phrase on scrappy bits of paper, shortly will give way to miniature electronic recording devices on which we will be able to note the time, amount, and intensity of the relevant behaviour or experience (e.g. the duration, intensity, and quality of head pain). Hence, the quality and range of the information on which psychologists base their advice and actions will undergo an astonishing transformation within the next few years.

This and other relevant data can be stored by patient or psychologist for as long as necessary. There will be almost no limit to the amount of available, accessible, manipulable data. Imagine how this will transform the nature of memorial problems. Patients whose powers of recognition and recall are failing will be provided with prosthetic memory devices that are programmed with all of the key biographical, social, and day-to-day information which the person might require. All that will be necessary is for the patient to push the relevant buttons — and if his power to execute even this simple action is faulty, it will be easy to install automatic signalling devices that present information at prearranged times or signals. Such prosthetic memory devices and other psychological aids will become as commonplace as spectacles. Prosthetic devices will place psychologists in a position to provide rehabilitation services on a scale of a kind that could not be contemplated as little as five years ago. Incidentally, if the early promise of cognitive therapy is fulfilled, it should be possible to programme into a miniature device the kinds of information that the depressed patient should have access to — instead of relying on his incomplete and often biased associative networks.

Other electronic devices will put at our disposal, in an easily accessible form, the banks of information which psychologists and others have collected during the past 20 to 30 years. It will be possible to call up a reference, and the detailed results reported in some distant part of the world, merely by tapping out the relevant code on your miniature reading screen. To some extent, the conflict of statistical versus clinical prediction will be resolved.

What then should psychologists look forward to and what should they promote? As far as the scope of clinical psychology is concerned, the expansion of the profession to include medical and health specialities additional to psychiatry is already underway, but needs to be accelerated. This wholly desirable and belated development has not yet advanced past the point of lame promises. A period of practical accomplishment is necessary. The provision of wider services will demand a considerable expansion of our teaching programmes, and students of clinical psychology will need to know a great deal more about anatomy, physiology, pathology, epidemiology, and so forth. All going well, the syllabus for students of clinical psychology in 1990 will be unrecognizable to today's teachers and students.

# Preface

The aim of the book is to describe and explain the expanding role and practice of clinical psychology within the National Health Service. The emphasis is on the wider aspect of the clinical psychologist's activities rather than on details relating to specific techniques and procedures.

In Great Britain, clinical psychologists began to function in hospitals as psychometricians ancillary to psychiatrists. However, with the increased recognition of the importance of psychological factors contributing to both mental and physical illness and the refinement of psychological methods of treatment, their role has rapidly expanded. The publication of the Trethowan Report in 1977 on *The Role of Psychologists in the Health Services* by the Department of Health and Social Security is widely acknowledged to be a landmark in the development of the profession. Its main recommendations strengthened the sense of purpose and identity which had begun to develop in the 1960s. In particular, it encouraged clinical psychologists throughout the country to organize themselves to act in a corporate manner and to diversify their professional activities.

The contributors are practising clinical psychologists who have described their practice in the post-Trethowan era and the characteristics of the settings in which they operate. The work is divided into four parts: Part I gives the general background relating to the development and management of the profession; Part II describes current practice in settings which were first to employ clinical psychologists; Part III relates to the expansion of services to client groups which have been specifically singled out in the Trethowan recommendations; Part IV concludes by giving overviews of professional developments in other European countries and in the United States of America.

ANDRÉE LIDDELL
*London, August 1982*

*PART I*

# Professional Organization

The Practice of Clinical Psychology in Great Britain
Edited by A. Liddell


*Chapter 1*

# *Professional development*

*Andrée Liddell*

## EARLY DEVELOPMENT

The early development of the practice of clinical psychology was as much tied to the Child Guidance movement in this country as it was in the United States of America (see Chapter 15). In the early days, the American contribution was more than just theoretical. Training and financial resources were granted to British psychologists and other staff from The New Commonwealth Fund of America. Funds were made available to set up a training clinic to demonstrate the new methods and to provide grants for psychologists and psychiatrists to study and practise in association with social workers who were following a further course in mental health work (Davidson, 1953; de Monchaux and Keir, 1961).

The Child Guidance movement originated in America as a new approach to the treatment of juvenile delinquency but it was rapidly expanded between the World Wars to help with a wide range of problem behaviour in children encountered at home or in school and referred to clinics established both in the community and in hospitals. Child Guidance clinics fostered a multidisciplinary team approach to the assessment, understanding, and treatment of presented problems; the team included a psychiatrist, an educational psychologist, and a social worker. In the classic model, each member of the team was expected to carry out separate and identifiable functions under the leadership of the psychiatrist. The psychologist's functions were regarded largely as those relating to assessment but included also play observation and remedial education. However, more varied partnerships, for example with paediatricians and speech therapists, developed and educational psychologists' contribution came to include, in addition to psychometrics, both interpretative and advisory aspects. In the mid-1930s employment prospects for these trainees were not good and the growth of the new child guidance service was very slow. Employing authorities saw the appointment of a multidisciplinary team as unnecessary for coping with the general run of problems about which teachers, for example, sought help. Consequently, educational psychologists alone of the three disciplines were sometimes employed by Local Education Authorities and before the passing of the 1944 Education Act the seeds were sown for School Psychological Services (Sampson, 1980).

Meanwhile, other psychologists had gradually begun to apply psychology initially in the form of research and subsequently to problems in mental illness and mental handicap hospitals. These psychologists were referred to from the start as *clinical psychologists* and many of their activities were carried out on a voluntary or part-time basis until the institution of the National Health Service in 1948 which greatly expanded the facilities of psychiatric out-patients' department and mental illness hospitals among other settings likely to require them. Psychiatrists working with adult patients had not been slow to show interest in the development and application of psychological assessment, especially in the field of mental subnormality. However, it was the Second World War which provided the opportunity for increased contact between psychologists and psychiatrists and they were seen to collaborate profitably in many areas, particularly in personnel selection for the Armed Forces, in addition to psychiatric casualties. This collaboration was preserved and extended during the post-war period in the National Health Service (Zangwill, 1966; Davis, 1974).

Although clinical psychologists in Great Britain were from the start greatly influenced by their American counterparts, they nevertheless developed a characteristic identity which resulted from their relationship, on one hand, with the British Psychological Society and, on the other, the National Health Service. The nature of these major influences will be discussed below followed by an appreciation of the trends of the last twenty years or so, taking the 1960s as the turning point which led to the coming of age of clinical psychology in this country.

## The British Psychological Society

The Psychological Society was founded in 1901 but changed its name to 'The British Psychological Society' in 1906. The composition of its founding members may seem strange to the present day psychologist since formal training in those days was not available. They were ten in number and included an experimental physiologist, a psychiatrist, a teacher, a lawyer, and others with a medical or philosophical background. The Society remained a relatively small and rather select group of people reporting their psychological experiments to each other until 1918 when it was decided to admit, as members, people interested in psychology as well as those actively engaged in psychological work. It continued to evolve over the years to accommodate the interests and needs of its growing and diverse membership as well as pressures from outside (Edgell, 1947, 1961; Knight, 1961). With the opening up of the Society to a wider membership, came the introduction of sections which were to cater for different interest groups. The first sections to be formed in this way were medical, educational, and industrial sections reflecting a strong interest in the applied fields. While the education section initially attracted the largest membership, the medical section was a close second. In 1941 the Society was incorporated under the Companies Act of 1929 and, in 1965, it received a Royal Charter. Probably the most far-reaching resolution for professional psychologists was passed in 1981 at the Annual General Meeting of the Society regarding the acceptance, in principle, of establishing a legal register of psychologists in the UK.

The idea of establishing a professional register for trained psychologists was not a new one. Hand in hand with the development of 'mental testing' came an awareness of its potential danger in untrained hands and a Professional Status Committee was set up in 1934 to inquire into the problem. With the incorporation of the Society in 1941, the Fellowship and the Associateship were introduced to differentiate members who were suitably trained and had worked in an acknowledged field of psychology. After 1958 every new Member of the Society needed to possess a university degree or postgraduate qualification in psychology.

Under the BPS umbrella, professional psychologists employed in Child Guidance and the Education Services were the first professionals to form a committee in 1943 (Committee of Professional Psychologists — Mental Health); clinical psychologists as they became established were admitted to this committee. In 1950 this group became a subsection called the Adult Section which aimed to cater for their special needs (Rawlings, 1951). New articles and byelaws of the Society were published in 1958 bringing into being the formation of an English Division of Professional Psychologists (Educational and Clinical). This was also approved in Scotland. The original Committee of Professional Psychologists was thus converted into divisions having made considerable advances in its endeavour to foster training and standards of practice for educational and clinical psychologists. Between 1945 and 1955, the membership of the Committee of Professional Psychologists had increased from 77 to 350. At the occasion of the Diamond Jubilee of the Society, Knight (1961) spoke of the above professional groups in the following way:

> These Divisions, and the Committee out of which they grew, have rendered very valuable services to their members, to the Society, to psychology and to the general public. They have helped to carry out one of the chief objects of the Society, which is 'to promote the efficiency and usefulness of its members by setting a high standard of professional education and knowledge and by compelling the observance of strict rules of professional conduct as a condition of membership or otherwise' (Article 3). They have kept a watchful eye on the conditions under which psychologists are employed and, for example have sought to preserve the independence of psychology in the medical field, where the clinical psychologist is regarded not as a mere medical auxiliary, but as providing a service parallel to that provided by hospital departments of physics or biochemistry (p. 29).

In 1966 the formation of a separate Division of Clinical Psychology comprising existing members of the Adult Section was approved by the Society. Its main aims were described in the following way in a contemporary issue of the *Bulletin* of the BPS:

> A major purpose in forming the Division of Clinical Psychology was to provide an organization within the structure of the British Psychological Society that could deal quickly with professional matters concerning clinical psychologists employed by the National Health Service, other than the trade-union matters falling within the sphere of the Association of Scientific Workers. Linked with this purpose was a strong wish that the executive body of the organization should have close and continuous contact with clinical psychologists working in the various National Health Service Regions. The Division of Clinical Psychology therefore is closely related to all its functions and activities in the National Health Service. This particularly applies to the conditions of training and employment required for membership and affiliate membership of the Division, the principles of representation on the Division Committee, the local organization of the Division and the Newsletter which will be a vehicle of communication between the Division Committee and the Regional Branches or Groups of the Division (Procter *et al.*, 1967, p. 28).

Between the inception of the separate Division of Clinical Psychology and 1980, there was a threefold increase of its membership making it the largest division approximating 10 per cent of the total membership of the BPS which was then 9,208 members.

At the end of 1973 the Council of the Society appointed two separate Boards to help co-ordinate its various activities especially those carried out by its sections (Scientific Affairs Board) and those of its divisions (Professional Affairs Board). This step in the reorganization of the BPS had been delayed until the appointment of the first full-time Secretary-General, Dr Ralph Hetherington.

The growing influence of the British Psychological Society on matters of public concern made itself felt particularly after its incorporation under the Companies Act in 1941, with further advances after it was granted a Royal Charter in 1965. Knight (1961) commenting on its services to the public during the period 1941–1961 listed the following contributions:

> it [the Society] investigated and published its findings on such matters of public concern as selection for secondary schools (1957). It has submitted expert and detailed evidence to various Departmental and Interdepartmental Committees and to a Royal Commission on such matters as: maladjusted children (1951); the training of teachers for work with handicapped children (1952); the law relating to mental illness and mental deficiency (1954); the law relating to homosexuality and prostitution (1955); the Home Office's concern with children and young persons (1958); the report of the Royal Commission on mental illness and mental deficiency (1958); the Mental Health Bill (1959); the training of staff of training centres for the mentally subnormal (1960); and drug addiction (1961) (p. 37).

BPS nominees or representatives have continued to be appointed to sit on or submit evidence to innumerable national and international committees such as the Parliamentary and Scientific Committee, the Mental Health Advisory Committee, the Royal Commission on the Health Service, the Royal Commission on Medical Education, Patients First, the Council of Europe, and Committees of the World Health Organization. It is obvious that in making many of the above contributions, the Society has had to draw directly on the expertise of its 'health' professionals.

**Clinical Psychologists in the National Health Service**

Shortly before the National Health Service came into being a blueprint was circulated regarding the personnel likely to be employed and the machinery for negotiating their salaries. But psychologists were not mentioned. Fortunately this blueprint came to the notice of the Society. Thanks to its intervention a career structure for psychologists was developed within the NHS. In fact, up to the present day the great majority of clinical psychologists are employed within the Service.

The National Health Service was inaugurated in 1948 by the National Health Service Acts of 1946 and 1947. Since the practice of clinical psychology in Great Britain has evolved almost exclusively within the NHS, an understanding of its structure is necessary to appreciate the position of its psychologists. Summerfield (1958) gave a clear and comprehensive exposition of the early organization of the Service with details of the employment conditions of the psychologists working in it during the first ten years of its existence. The first Whitley circular detailing qualifications and conditions of service for psychologists in the NHS appeared in 1952 (PTA circulars 10 and 14). Within the Whitley machinery clinical psychologists come under the Professional and Technical Whitley Council 'A' along with other non-medical graduate scientists such as physicists and biochemists. The basic qualification which has remained unchanged to the present day is an honours degree in psychology from a British university or other equivalent qualification approved by the Minister of Health or Secretary of State for Scotland. In addition to the degree in psychology, a period of postgraduate training was specified although this period of training has increased from one year to three years over the last thirty years (see Chapter 2). The grading structure of the first circular consisted of four psychologist grades: (1) *assistant psychologist* for those who served one year of training under a Senior or had followed a recognized training course, (2) *psychologist*, who were aged 25 years or more in addition to postgraduate training, (3) *senior psychologist* whose function might be to supervise others, and (4) *top grade psychologist* for 'special posts'; the establishment of such posts was subject to the approval of the Minister of Health or Secretary of State for Scotland. Conditions of service were left vague with hours unspecified and mention only that the appointed psychologist was to carry out the proper performance of the job.

Other PTA circulars followed modifying the original grading structure in terms of training, responsibilities, and salaries. For example, a probationary period of three years was required before promotion to the basic grade of psychologist (PTA circular 27 in 1954) but this period was shortened for those who had followed a formal postgraduate training course (PTA circular 39 in 1956). The first list of NHS approved training courses for clinical psychologists appeared in 1957 in PTA circular 52 and included one course in an academic institution (the Institute of Psychiatry, London) and two non-institution based courses (the Adult Department of the Tavistock Clinic, London and the Crichton Royal Hospital, Dumfries). These courses represented different approaches and bases for the practice of clinical psychology establishing it on a recognizably broad conceptual basis. Hetherington (1981) attributed great benefits for the profession from the internal 'creative tensions' generated in the early days by these competing approaches. Probably the most important change in the grading structure occurred with PTA circular 72 in 1959. This circular introduced the *principal grade* (between senior and top grades) for a post with considerable responsibilities and normally given to someone in charge of psychological services at an institution.

It should be added that over those years the BPS was increasingly consulted regarding the vetting of qualifications of applications to NHS psychologists posts, recognition of new training courses, and the appointment of psychologists as advisers within the DHSS. In 1982 further major redifinitions occurred for the principal and top grades — the latter being subdivided into two levels. In these latest definitions, responsibility for the management of psychologists and their services was firmly placed on the individuals concerned.

## DEVELOPMENTS FROM THE 1960s ONWARDS

Several factors contributed to the coming of age of clinical psychology in Great Britain. Some of them already mentioned above related directly to the growing number and expanding activities of its practitioners which in turn resulted in changed self-perceptions emerging into a strong sense of identity. Other factors were less direct and related to the greater acceptability of psychological explanations and interventions by an increasing number of other professionals who had studied psychology as part of their training as well as by the general public. With a greater sense of identity and purpose, clinical psychologists found themselves better able to organize themselves to alter their positions *vis-à-vis* the BPS, the NHS, and the public at large.

Davis (1974), taking a historical perspective of clinical psychology in this country, identified some of the major social changes during the decade immediately preceding his publication. He noted that clinical psychologists had been increasingly using the *Bulletin* of the Society to air questions affecting their profession. He also remarked on a new spirit of acceptance and tolerance experienced by clinical psychologists in the NHS which led to the creation of new posts and improved career prospects. These trends appeared to interact with an increasing demand for places on postgraduate training programmes in clinical psychology among psychology graduates. Another reason to explain this preference was given by Davis as clinical psychology 'offering careers consistent with the value-system and aspirations of a high proportion of psychology graduates' (p. 135). In any case the rush for training places in clinical psychology provided the impetus for the expansion and regulation of training (see Chapter 2) and the result was that some of the most able graduates in the country became available to fulfil the manpower needs of the NHS.

Above and beyond the organizational issues, much in evidence in contemporary debates, issues relating to role and function were also hotly pursued. The recognition of psychological treatment being carried out by psychologists was firmly established in the 1960s. The growth of interest in behaviour therapy greatly accelerated this change along with a willingness to conceptualize problems encountered among patients and clients in psychological rather than psychiatric terms (see Chapter 5). This led to an appreciation of the psychologist's contribution outside psychiatry (Gwynne Jones, 1969; Dabbs, 1972; Eysenck and Rachman, 1973; Davis, 1974; Graham, 1977; Hetherington, 1981; Pond, 1982).

Two separate reports from the Department of Health and Social Security are considered to be of importance in determining the fortunes of clinical psychologists in the NHS. The first of these was from a committee chaired by Sir Solly Zuckerman (Zuckerman, 1968); its importance rested in the fact that it failed to include psychologists in its recommendations, but this led to the second report from a sub-committee under the chairmanship of Professor W. H. Trethowan which focused exclusively on the role of psychologists in the Health Services (Trethowan, 1977).

*Zuckerman Committee.* The terms of reference of the Committee were: 'To consider the future organization and development of hospital Scientific and Technical Services in National Health Service hospitals and the broad pattern of staffing required and to make recommendations' (Zuckerman, 1968, p. iii). At the time the job description of clinical psychologists was made in the following manner:

> Clinical psychologists in the hospital service are employed in psychiatric hospitals, hospitals for the mentally subnormal and out-patients departments dealing with adults and children. They carry out tests of intelligence, temperament, personality, deterioration and aptitudes in order to help psychiatrists in diagnosis, treatment and vocational guidance. They may also undertake teaching and training and participate in development and research relating to psychological problems (Zuckerman, 1968, p. 52).

The Committee started its work at a time when psychologists were inclined to emphasize their scientific rather than their clinical role. However, the Committee's recommendations did not become mandatory until 1971 when clinical psychologists' opinion had swung in favour of wanting to be regarded as *clinicians* having a primary function in treatment not assessment though, at the same time, accepting their function as applied scientists and their role in teaching, multidisciplinary team work and research.

*Trethowan Sub-Committee.* The Zuckerman Committee's recommendation that clinical psychologists should be reviewed further led directly to the appointment of the Trethowan Sub-Committee by the Standing Mental Health Advisory Committee. Clinical psychologists were well represented on the sub-committee in the persons of Professor A. D. B. Clarke, Miss May Davidson, and Professor H. Gwynne Jones. The sub-committee started its work at the end of 1972 but did not actually report until 1977. During that time a large number of organizations and individuals submitted evidence.

Broadly speaking the issues considered by the sub-committee related to, (a) *what* clinical psychologists could do, to *whom* and *where*, (b) their relationship with other health professionals including questions relating to referral sources and responsibility, and (c) organization of psychological services, levels of staffing (including the employment of technicians), career structure, and training. Their main conclusions were that clinical psychologists have a contribution to make in many fields of health care though their role had been restricted due, in part, to their small numbers. Major fields of application were listed as mental illness, mental handicap, physical handicap, child and adolescent health problems, neurology, general medicine, geriatrics, community medicine, and general medical practice. Recommendation was made that full professional status be accorded to clinical psychologists in the NHS with the proviso that medical responsibility for treatment cannot be handed over to any other profession in the Service. This made some form of medical cover a necessity and 'responsibility' a broad concept in need of further definition for operational purposes. A multidisciplinary team approach was advocated for psychologists and the members of other health service professions. Area Psychological Services were recommended as the appropriate structure to be managed by psychologists of principal status or above, preferably associated with a district general hospital. Research and a contribution to the training of other professions by clinical psychologists were especially mentioned as valuable activities to be encouraged. It was further recommended that Regional Psychological Advisory Committees be established and that they be given recognition by the Secretaries of State. In addition, mention was made that Regional Health Authorities should be involved in appointments at area level to posts graded principal psychologist (and above) and that they have an overall responsibility in promoting training. It was further recommended that all clinical psychologists should be required to obtain a formal postgraduate qualification and that the DHSS should consider financing training courses. In relation to staffing and career structure, an annual increase of 80 psychologists was envisaged in the light of existing and planned training facilities resulting in some 1,100 psychologists in six or seven years (that is by 1984), this being regarded as a minimum target. Recommendations were made for clinical psychologists to be supported by psychological technicians and for the establishment of a new grade of senior principal psychologist between the existing principal and top grades. The greatest unmet needs were identified as being in the fields of child psychiatry and mental handicap and it was thought desirable that clinical psychologists should become more closely involved in the primary care setting with general practitioners. Finally, it was recommended that a full-time psychologist be appointed centrally to the Department of Health and Social Security with responsibilities for the development of the service nationally.

Approximately five years had elapsed between the setting up of the Trethowan Sub-Committee and the publication of its report (Trethowan, 1977) with the accompanying DHSS circular introducing the main structural changes. These five years were characterized by important national changes. In 1974, the NHS underwent the first major reorganization since its inception in 1948 and it was thought that the upheaval it caused was instrumental in postponing the publication of the Trethowan findings. There is no doubt that the circulation, in March 1974, of the consultative document of the sub-committee alarmed reactionary forces within the medical profession. Be that as it may, it was nevertheless submitted to the Secretary of State in June 1975 but did not appear officially until May 1977. However, many clinical psychologists greatly encouraged by the consultative document, had meanwhile fostered as far as possible, the changes which they expected to be made formally and by the time the report was published it did not appear particularly revolutionary to anyone concerned. Unfortunately the economic climate had worsened to a degree which prohibited the implementation of many of the recommendations, for instance, the appointment of a full-time psychologist who would have co-ordinated psychological services nationally.

Five years after the appearance of the Trethowan Report, clinical psychologists found themselves numerically in excess of the manpower predictions that were made for six or seven years hence and facing yet another reorganization of the NHS. Areas were abolished in April 1982, leaving staff with districts to organize — a level preferred by many of them (see Chapter 4). Services outside usual settings were developing gradually (see Part III). Training facilities had been extended to almost every Region in the country and the number and calibre of applicants for postgraduate courses had remained high. Formal postgraduate qualifications had been made compulsory for probationary practice in the NHS and a new top grade level post had been added to discriminate between carrying different levels of responsibility. NHS psychologists had developed the practice of meeting regularly at district, area, or regional levels and found support and guidance from peer groups. This undoubtedly fostered in them a greater sense of identity and confidence than they had experienced in the past. In spite of the fact that the committees they formed in the NHS were not yet recognized as originally recommended, many of them were approached by administrators for advice. Without minimizing the problems anticipated through reorganization and the severe financial stringencies, clinical psychologists were nevertheless experiencing a greater sense of fulfilment and optimism than at any other time in their short history.

## REFERENCES

Dabbs, A. R. (1972). The changing role of clinical psychologists in the National Health

Service. *Bulletin of The British Psychological Society,* **25**, 107–109.

Davidson, M. A. (1953). Current trends in clinical psychology. In C. A. Mace and P. E. Vernon (eds), *Current Trends in British Psychology*. London: Methuen.

Davis, H. (1974). Clinical psychology: A historical perspective. *Bulletin of The British Psychological Society,* **27**, 135–139.

de Monchaux, C., and Keir, G. H. (1961). British psychology 1945–1957. *Acta Psychologica,* **18**, 120–180.

Edgell, B. (1947). British Psychological Society. *British Journal of Psychology,* **37**, 113–132.

Edgell, B. (1961). The British Psychological Society 1901–1941. In H. Steinberg (ed.), *The British Psychological Society 1901–1961*. London: BPS.

Eysenck, H. J. and Rachman, S. (1973). The future of clinical psychology. *Bulletin of The British Psychological Society,* **26**, 113–116.

Gwynne Jones, H. (1969). Clinical psychology. In B.M. Foss (ed.), *Supplement to the Bulletin of The British Psychological Society on the occasion of the International Congress of Psychology, London, 1969.* London: BPS.

Graham, P. (1977). Psychology and psychiatry — relations and overlap. *Bulletin of The British Psychological Society,* **30**, 76–79.

Hetherington, R. (1981). The changing role of the clinical psychologist. *Bulletin of The British Psychological Society,* **34**, 12–14.

Knight, R. (1961). The Society since 1941. In H. Steinberg (ed.), *The British Psychological Society 1901–1961.* London: BPS.

Pond, D. (1982). Psychology — prop or profession? *Bulletin of The British Psychological Society,* **35**, 49–55.

Procter, M., Roe, A. M., Desai, M. M. and Robertson, J. P. J. (1967). Membership of a division. *Bulletin of The British Psychological Society,* **20**, 28–29.

Rawlings, G. (1951). Committee of Professional Psychologists (Mental Health). *Quarterly Bulletin of The British Psychological Society,* **2**, 75–78.

Sampson, O. (1980). *Child Guidance: Its History, Provenance and Future*. Leicester: BPS.

Summerfield, A. (1958). Clinical psychology in Britain. *American Psychologist,* **13**, 171–176.

Trethowan, W. H. (1977). *The Role of Psychologists in the Health Services*. London: HMSO.

Zangwill, O. L. (1966). In defence of clinical psychology. *Bulletin of The British Psychological Society,* **19**, 13–21.

Zuckerman, S. (1968). *Hospital Scientific and Technical Services*. London: HMSO.

The Practice of Clinical Psychology in Great Britain
Edited by A. Liddell


*Chapter 2*

# *The training and function of a clinical psychologist*

*Andrée Liddell*

This chapter will deal first with the development of postgraduate training courses in clinical psychology offered in this country. Secondly, the main functions of the clinical psychologist will be explained in relation to training.

## TRAINING COURSES

Clinical psychologists in the UK are university graduates in psychology (honours degree or equivalent) who have followed a postgraduate programme of studies in which they have learnt to apply the principles of psychology to various problems encountered in a variety of clinical settings. Formally organized training and accreditation of relevant courses of study by the British Psychological Society evolved slowly.

The first formal postgraduate course was started in 1947 at the Maudsley Hospital. From 1947 to 1966 the Maudsley offered a 13-month training for which a diploma was awarded; in 1966 it became a two-year course and a Master's degree of the University of London was awarded as the programme then came under a constituent Institute of the University — the Institute of Psychiatry. It was not until the 1960s that other Master's courses were developed at Belfast, Liverpool, Glasgow, Leeds, Newcastle, Edinburgh, and Birmingham universities. In the 1970s other two-year postgraduate courses in clinical psychology were started at Surrey, Manchester, and Aberdeen universities while, at the North East London Polytechnic and Exeter University, the training period was extended to three years still culminating in a Master's degree. In 1976, a two-tiered mode of training began at Birmingham University — two years to an M.Sc. degree with two additional years for a Ph.D for selected candidates already on their Master's course. In 1982 another three-year course was started at Leicester University and a two-year course at the Plymouth Polytechnic. Lively discussions in other parts of the country were also taking place regarding new establishments. The majority of Master's courses in clinical psychology are now in academic departments of psychology while those which are not are either in departments of psychiatry or the joint responsibility of both the departments of psychiatry and psychology of their respective universities.

Presently, most postgraduate courses are based in academic institutions. However, an earlier form of NHS in-service training has undergone several refinements and is now receiving formal approval from the British Psychological Society and recognition by the DHSS. Since 1968 the Society has awarded a national diploma to in-service trainees after they have followed a systematic programme of training accredited on the same criteria as institution-based courses and passed the examinations conducted by the Society.

In-service training developed alongside the National Health Service and was, for a considerable period of time, an alternative form of training to help supply the requisite of clinical psychologists. In its earliest form, it comprised a three-year apprenticeship, usually in a psychiatric hospital, under the guidance of a trained clinical psychologist of at least senior status. *Ad hoc* and then more formal in-service schemes were developed as a result of BPS initiatives to facilitate training outside academic institutions. With the inception of a BPS Diploma in clinical psychology candidates who wished to take the examination were required to have experience with a variety of problems, for example, mental handicap, child and adolescent psychological problems, and adult psychological problems. These NHS in-service courses now have organizers especially appointed at regional level to arrange programmes of study and co-ordinate practical placements. With the formal recognition which the BPS now accords to courses approved by its assessment panels they are accepted by the Whitley Council as an equivalent form of training to university or polytechnic based courses.

If the two methods of training described above are combined, 157 new trainees were admitted in 1980; between one in four and one in five applicants having obtained places on approved courses (Clearing House for Post-Graduate Courses in Clinical Psychology, 1981 Report). It is estimated that keeping intake of trainees relatively constant would result in a yearly growth of approximately 8 per cent of qualified clinical psychologists (Kat, 1980). The profession is unanimous in viewing, as the most important single development, the long overdue decision of the Whitley Council in 1981 to make a formal postgraduate qualification (Master's Degree or BPS Diploma) an obligatory condition for the appointment of clinical psychologists at the Basic Grade in the NHS.

## Criteria for Approval of Courses by the British Psychological Society

The BPS Committee on Training in Clinical Psychology operates on behalf of the Professional Affairs Board and the Division of Clinical Psychology. The Committee is made up of representatives of various parties which have particular interest and skill in training, for instance, the Committee of University Clinical Psychology Training Courses (representing institution based courses), the Committee of Organizers of Regional In-Service Courses in Clinical

Psychology (representing NHS based courses), and the Board of Examiners for the British Psychological Society's Diploma in Clinical Psychology. The terms of reference of the Committee are thus:

(a) To promote and ensure high standards of training in professional practice in clinical psychology;
(b) To review and monitor the standards of training in clinical psychology at all levels;
(c) To provide reports and recommendations relating to the standards of training in clinical psychology at all levels;
(d) To transact such business as may be referred to the Committee by the Professional Affairs Board or the Division of Clinical Psychology. (BPS Committee on Training in Clinical Psychology, Constitution 1981.)

It may seem strange to clinical psychologists outside Britain to read from the relevant document relating to criteria for approval that clinical psychologists are specifically trained for employment in the NHS. The aims of training were recently restated as:

> Courses should aim to meet the requirements of a professional training in clinical psychology as formulated by the Committee on Training in Clinical Psychology, and with due regard to the current Whitley Council agreements. They should be designed to provide trainees with a general training including a wide variety of experience and range of clinical skills which may be required by a Basic Grade (post-probationary) clinical psychologist in the NHS. (BPS: Professional Affairs Board, 1982).

The acknowledged aim of training is to produce a psychologist able to fulfil the role envisaged in the Trethowan Report of 1977 'in many fields of health care'. With this in view the trainees are given experience with clients of all age groups in different fields of health care making their training comprehensive and generic in its early phases. The areas of psychologists' functioning listed in the 1979 BPS *Criteria for the Assessment of Post Graduate Training Courses in Clinical Psychology* (and implied in the redraft of 1982) are:

(i) Assessment
(ii) Treatment, behaviour modification, and rehabilitation
(iii) Research
(iv) Communication with other professional groups and hospital departments, including experience of teaching
(v) Professional conduct
(vi) Management and organization of health services

These areas will be examined in some detail in the next section.

The BPS also requires that course, wherever sited, be managed by practising clinical psychologists and that there be close collaboration at all levels between clinical supervisors, academic tutors, and their trainees. This often onerous involvement by NHS practitioners provides a valuable incentive for the updating of people whose training is now outmoded and keeps staff abreast of new developments. It also stops academics from building 'ivory towers' and keeps training realistic and sensitive to current demands. These features of our training may have provided more cohesion in the philosophy which guided its development than is apparent in other countries where differing models of training are often in conflict (see Chapter 15). However, it would also be wrong to imply that we have achieved perfect harmony and uniformity. Concern is occasionally voiced regarding standardization of clinical experience (Hallam and Liddell, 1978) and suspicions regarding clinical psychologists in academe are openly admitted by NHS clinicians (Dry, 1981).

### Centralization of Applications to Courses and Characteristics of Applicants

In 1980, a Clearing House for postgraduate courses in clinical psychology was set up at Birmingham University. It operates on a model similar to that already familiar and long established by universities in this country for their undergraduate courses (UCCA) and by institutions offering Social Work courses (CCTESW). Details of clinical psychology courses are printed annually in a handbook which applicants can study before placing their application with the Clearing House which in turn distributes these applications to course centres. It also offers a pool system where candidates who were not offered a place by any of the centres of their choice are recirculated to centres who have unfilled places. Details of courses are made available in late summer/early autumn preceding the year of intake.

Applicants to the North East London Polytechnic course were studied over two separate intakes preceding the establishment of the Clearing House when it was common for candidates to apply separately to several courses offered at that time (Liddell and Boyle, 1980). Therefore, some degree of generalization of the results may be warranted. Applications to both intakes were similar in that women were somewhat in excess of men, and the majority of applicants had obtained 'relevant' experience along the lines suggested in the *Clearing House Handbook*. There was no sex difference in either quality of degree or experience and the means of the ages of all applicants of both intake groups was 26 years.

## MAIN FUNCTIONS OF CLINICAL PSYCHOLOGISTS

The resolution passed at the Annual Conference of the British Psychological Society of 1981 regarding the acceptance in principle of the setting up of a Legal Register of Psychologists in the UK was greatly welcomed by clinical psychologists. For one thing, they find themselves the only unregistered professional group in the NHS (Watts, 1980) and very much behind, in this respect, their colleagues in America and some other European countries (see Chapters 14 and 15). At this stage, the proposal accepted was to consider a general register of all psychologists by an Act of Parliament. Unfortunately this type of register would not differentiate between applied psychologists such as clinical psychologists and other psychologists whose training was primarily theoretical.

Dörken (1976) explained the distinction between licensing and certifying of psychologists in the USA. In that country psychologists operate under one or the other type of legislation depending on the state in which they practise. Laws relating to licensing attempt to seek to define the practice of psychology but restrict certain functions to psychologists and other professionals if trained to carry out these functions. Certification, on the other hand, protects the title *psychologist* and only qualified psychologists are entitled to use it. Certification is more in the nature of registration as sought by British psychologists. It is not as easy to differentiate and define the skills which clinical psychologists offer health care as it is, for instance, to characterize the functions of dentists or opticians. Also psychological methods are used by other professionals in the Health Services. However, carried out by psychologists they can be said to vary in terms of approach and emphasis. The professional psychologist's background of theoretical knowledge and broader experience in its application influences the choice of method he/she makes. This choice can be said to be made with greater flexibility and appreciation of scientific findings than can be achieved without a clinical psychologist training. The functions of assessment, therapy, and research will be focused on from the clinical psychologist's perspective; issues relating to communication, conduct and management will be discussed subsequently.

**Assessment**

Of all the skills offered by clinical psychologists practices relating to psychological assessment have most often been criticized inside as well as outside the profession. White (1972) deplored the fact that, some 50 years ago, clinical psychologists had chosen from psychology what he viewed as the two 'weakest boxes of psychological tools' — *psychometrics* and *psychotherapy* — and that both practices were genereally unrelated to each other. However, he acknowledged the contribution of psychometric methods to personnel selection and training during the Second World War and advocated a wider interactional approach to human measurement to be applied in a wider variety of settings. Smail (1973) suspected that clinical psychologists eased themselves into the NHS as 'scientific testers' a role which was too literally taken and resulted in their being eventually perceived as 'analogous to pathology laboratory technicians'. On the other hand, it is precisely the psychologist's evaluative approach to assessment which has made this role untenable.

*Psychometrics*. Drever (1973) defined *psychometrics* as: 'mathematical or measurement aspects of psychological experiments; more recently, statistical treatment of mental test results'. It is with the latter and narrower definition that psychologists in the NHS first made their mark for better or for worse. Within psychology, principles of test construction had been developed for the measurement of psychological functions and functioning. These principles dictated strict criteria for the establishment of the reliability and validity of such measures which had to be tested on representative samples of the population they were said to represent. Undeniable success, in terms of predictive value, was attached to the measurement of certain well defined characteristics such as intelligence and occupational skills. On the other hand, diagnosis of psychiatric conditions was not so easily quantifiable (Goldberg, 1974; Horn, 1976; Weiss and Davison, 1981).

Clinical psychologists were repeatedly provided with the evidence that human nature is infinitely complex and variable and that the haphazard rating of dogmatically selected attributes did it less than justice and, in some instances, actually harmed the prospects of certain of their clients. For example, the knowledge of someone's IQ or that he was diagnosed as schizophrenic has little prognostic value unless other factors such as social context are considered; usually the aforementioned labels are not even closely related to treatment and management of the case. Therefore, in conscience, clinical psychologists are no longer willing to impart this type of information unless they are made aware of the use to be made of it. Furthermore, because of their knowledge of test construction and their training in the administration of standardized tests, they feel justified in reserving the right to determine for themselves the appropriateness of psychological testing for the same reasons they would not wish to influence their medical colleagues when they are prescribing some form of medication.

*Restriction of tests.* The effects of wrongly categorizing or mislabelling may not be as obvious as those of *thalidomide* to the unfortunate children damaged by the drug. Nevertheless, the restriction of particular psychological tests to those who are trained to administer them is an international practice.

In Great Britain, tests are largely distributed through the NFER-Nelson Publishing Company. The publisher is a department of the National Foundation for Education Research which is an independent organization 'devoted to progress in education'. Financing for the Foundation comes from Local Education Authorities, the Department of Education and Science as well as teachers' organizations and universities. Tests and related materials are distributed in accordance with a strict test qualification coding system recommended by the British Psychological Society. Under the system, named qualified individuals *only* are provided with certain tests.

*Other forms of assessment.* In addition to standardized tests of psychological functions and diagnostic assessments mentioned above, Trethowan (1977) reported two other broad categories of assessment identified by the BPS, namely, 'physiological measures used as indices of psychological functioning or change' and 'measurement procedures used to reflect the problems and progress of particular patients or groups of patients'. The Society emphasized the close relationship between assessment and therapy and the importance of assessment in choosing between alternative forms of treatment' (Section 4.11). To that end the clinical psychologist needs to become familiar and evaluate a quickly expanding technology relating to behavioural assessment (Ciminero *et al*., 1977; Hersen and Bellack, 1981). This technology has gone a long way in assisting the clinician with operationalizing goals for therapeutic interventions and monitoring resultant changes.

Evaluating in the broadest sense is primarily in the functioning of clinical psychologists. Going back to Drever's dictionary definition of psychometrics as 'mathematical or measurement aspects of psychological experiments', it can be said to embody the philosophy of the applied scientist as an implicit superordinate aim of training.

**Therapy**

The British Psychological Society suggested to the Trethowan Sub-Committee that 45 per cent of the clinical psychologist's time be spent in treatment and rehabilitation as compared to assessment and diagnosis (10%), research (20%), teaching (15%), administration, organizational work, and continuing professional training (10%) (Trethowan, 1977). Psychotherapy, or the treatment of disorders by psychological methods, as an area of functioning is not easy to encompass. Within psychology itself, models of man still compete with each other (Chapman and Jones, 1980) throwing perspectives on abnormal behaviour into conflict (Price, 1978). Therefore, psychotherapists of different persuasion are seen to operate under very different assumptions, adding a great deal of confusion to an already complicated situation. This type of situation cannot be said to be unique in the history of scientific endeavours. However, it produces a great deal of stress in those who cannot tolerate ambiguity, be they client or therapist!

*Orientation*. Approaches to psychotherapy are generally defined by Corsini (1979) and, more specifically, from the clinical psychologist's standpoint by Garfield (1975) and Bernstein and Nietzel (1980).

In 1978 the Division of Clinical Psychology of the BPS established a Working Party on Psychological Therapies which had, among its terms of reference, that of considering the state of training in psychological therapies in the United Kingdom as well as of considering the commonalities and divergences between various approaches to psychological treatment and also to review the present state of research in the psychological therapies (BPS: Division of Clinical Psychology, 1979).

This working party quoted a broad definition of *psychological therapies* from Meltzoff and Hornreich (1970):

> informed and planful application of techniques derived from established psychological principles, by persons qualified through training and experience to understand

these principles and to apply these techniques with the intention of assisting individuals to modify such personal characteristics as feelings, values, attitudes and behaviours which are judged by the therapist to be maladaptive or maladjustive (p. 6).

The above definition was thought to represent 'individual and group work cast within a wide range of theoretical frameworks, from the behavioural to the psychoanalytic' (I.7, BPS: Division of Clinical Psychology, 1979).

It was noted by the working party that psychodynamic theory and therapy had tended to develop outside the National Health Service and that major theoretical advances in this orientation had been due to psychoanalysts in the private sector, usually psychiatrists who saw psychoanalysis as their exclusive province. The following historical note was also found in the Report:

it was only with the development of such unequivocally psychological disciplines of theory and practice as the behaviour and client-centred approaches that clinical psychologists gained the secure right to practise psychological therapy within the NHS. These newer approaches were especially amenable to the research methodologies in which psychologists have special expertise. Although differences between the types of treatment espoused by the majority of clinical psychologists on the one hand and many psychiatrists on the other hand are still clearly identifiable — particularly since a greater proportion of psychiatrists have been trained within the broadly psychodynamic/object relations tradition as developed by the British Psychoanalytical Society and such institutions as the Tavistock Clinic and the Cassell Hospital — these differences appear to be diminishing at the present time. In retrospect, it now appears that the isolation of psychodynamic theory from the mainstream of psychology has worked to the disadvantage of both. Psychoanalytic theory is a psychological, not medical theory. Having now gained, via behavioural and client-centred methods, the acceptance of the psychologist's role in treatment (exemplified by the Trethowan Report) the time is now ripe for us to build and utilize the recognition that all psychological therapies depend upon psychological theories, rationales and methods' (VI.4, BPS: Division of Clinical Psychology, 1979).

All clinical psychology training courses were shown to offer training in behavioural methods (the only named method on the 1979 BPS Criteria for Approval). Some courses train exclusively within a behavioural training while others supplement their basic behavioural approach with other therapeutic approaches, duration of courses being an important factor in determining the extent and depth of coverage. However, it is evident that 'an ecletic but unified treatment of psychotherapeutic processes' such as that described by Garfield (1980) is gaining ground with British Psychologists (Pond, 1978). In addition there exists a small but increasing number of post-probationer therapy courses for qualified clinical psychologists who wish to extend their therapeutic skills. In 1981 the BPS began to vet post-probationer training courses along the same lines as basic training (BPS: Professional Affairs Board, 1981).

**Research**

Williams (1981) classified and listed the research dissertations of postgraduate students who were registered on approved courses in clinical psychology between 1977 and 1979. Over the three years under scrutiny, he reported on 271 theses; of these, the largest number presented were within the category of *behaviour modification, general hospital* (GP, surgical patients, etc.) was listed second. This undoubtedly reflected the behavioural orientation of most training courses and the general preoccupation of the profession to extend its activities outside psychiatry. It should also be noted that the areas of *mental handicap, neuropsychology*, and *geriatric psychology* were next in line. This is considered both surprising and heartening as these areas had been consistently chosen as least preferred by the applicants sampled by Liddell and Boyle (1980).

The contribution which clinical psychologists are making to research in the NHS is likely to be increasingly recognized and valued. Because there is a formal training programme in virtually all NHS regions, research by clinical psychologists is carried out (at least by trainees) on a regular basis throughout the country. To the trainees, it is an activity which is carried during the latter part of training when they have acquired an understanding of the methodology applicable and of the problems needing inquiry. Through their own projects, they are made aware that applying the principles of general psychology is not straightforward; they also learn to evaluate a rapidly expanding research literature which should be cautiously monitored before it is allowed to affect practice.

Support for the role of applied scientist has been regularly forthcoming from the profession (Davidson, 1977; Whitehead, 1978; Feldman, 1981) though disquiet has been voiced regarding the breadth of present day psychology as the basis for such application (Shapiro, 1975; Duckwork, 1981). There is no doubt that clinical psychologists will continue to influence psychology by providing hypotheses to be tested from clinical observations.

## Communication, Conduct, and Management

While clinical psychologists were seen as adjuncts in departments of psychiatry, they seemed to devote little time in considering issues relating to communications, conduct, and management. The low profile they kept occasioned a great deal of perceptual stress by all (including themselves) regarding their role and function as compared to those of psychiatrists.

From the earliest days, psychologists had been asked to teach their professional colleagues the basic principles of psychology. Their teaching was often criticized as being at too theoretical a level and made them appear as intelligent schizoids, having little relevant knowledge to offer. In fairness, this can be said to have reflected as much the crudeness of psychology as a basic science, as their inability to abstract relevant information. As psychology progressed and achieved greater applicability to shared problems, it became recognized as an important area of study for medical students, and other colleagues. Consequently lecturing posts in psychology were established in medical schools throughout the country and the services of psychologists requested in training schools for nurses, social workers, speech therapists, *et al*. This has resulted in more sophisticated and receptive medical and other colleagues on the one hand and, on the other, clinical psychologists who are tackling the issues relevant to communicating their knowledge and skills to achieve greater impact on all health services (Griffiths, 1976; Kent and Clarke, 1981; Vingoe, 1981).

The British Psychological Society circulated its first guidance for good practice in clinical psychology in the 1970s in preparation for a mandatory code of ethics (BPS: Division of Clinical Psychology, 1974). A revised version integrating recommendations from the membership is in preparation. One of the strongest of the recommendations for amendment came as a result of the *DCP Working Party on Psychological Therapies* and related to 'transmitting skills to others including non-professionals' (BPS: Division of Clinical Psychology, 1979). While it is impossible to restrict therapy in the same way as psychological standardized tests it is, nevertheless, believed that clinical psychologists should take on responsibility for seeing to the strict implementation and appropriateness of the therapeutic programmes they may teach others.

Management of clinical psychologists by clinical psychologists is now an accomplished fact (see Chapter 4). Usually they are no longer directly responsible to psychiatrists but are more likely to be found in departments of clinical psychology accountable to a District Management Team. This necessitates from them a greater understanding of the functioning of the National Health Service and its various agencies along with the managerial skills and foresight needed to maintain and develop realistic services.

In sum, British clinical psychologists are trained in the NHS as applied scientists to carry out responsibly a number of functions which are considered of benefit in various aspects of health care. These functions will be taken up again and expanded in the following chapters by practising psychologists who take their own settings as illustration.

## REFERENCES

British Psychological Society: Division of Clinical Psychology (1974). *Current Guidelines for the Professional Practice of Clinical Psychology*. Leicester: BPS.

British Psychological Society: Division of Clinical Psychology (1979). *Report of the Working Party on the Psychological Therapies.* Leicester: BPS.

British Psychological Society: Professional Affairs Board (1979). *Criteria for the Assessment of Post-graduate Training Courses in Clinical Psychology*. Leicester: BPS.

British Psychological Society: Professional Affairs Board (1981). Criteria for the assessment of post-qualification courses for applied psychologists in psychological therapy. *Bulletin of The British Psychological Society,* **34**, 130.

British Psychological Society: Professional Affairs Board (1982). *Criteria for the Assessment of Post-graduate Training Courses in Clinical Psychology* (draft). Leicester: BPS.

Bernstein, D., and Nietzel, M. T. (1980). *Introduction to Clinical Psychology*. New York: McGraw-Hill.
Chapman, A. J., and Jones, D. M. (eds) (1980). *Models of Man*. Leicester: BPS.
Ciminero, A. R., Calhoun, K. S., and Adams, H. E. (eds) (1977). *Handbook of Behavioural Assessment*. New York: John Wiley.
Corsini, R. (ed.) (1979). *Current Psychotherapies*, 2nd ed. Itasca: F. E. Peacock.
Davidson, M. (1977). The scientific/applied debate in psychology: A contribution. *Bulletin of The British Psychological Society,* **30**, 273–278.
Dörken, H. (ed.) (1976). *The Professional Psychologist Today*. San Francisco: Jossey-Bass.
Drever, J. (1973). *A Dictionary of Psychology*, rev. ed. Harmondsworth: Penguin.
Dry, A. (1981). Overlords or honoured guest — alternative models of NHS and university relationships. *Division of Clinical Psychology Newsletter,* **31**, 15–17.
Duckwork, D. H. (1981). Toward a psychological science that can be applied. *Bulletin of The British Psychological Society,* **34**, 237–240.
Feldman, M. P. (1981). The employment of clinical psychologists: present and future. In I. McPherson and A. Sutton, *Reconstructing Psychological Practice*. London: Croom Helm.
Garfield, S. L. (1975). *Clinical Psychology: The Study of Personality and Behaviour*. London: Edward Arnold.
Garfield, S. L. (1980). *Psychotherapy: An Ecletic Approach*. New York: John Wiley.
Goldberg, L. R. (1974). Objective diagnostic tests and measures. *Annual Review of Psychology,* **25**, 343–366.
Griffiths, R. D. P. (1976). The teaching of psychology in medical schools: A pat on the back or a kick in the pants? *Bulletin of The British Psychological Society,* **29**, 269–273.
Hallam, R. S., and Liddell, A. (1978). A community clinic for teaching psychotherapy. *Bulletin of The British Psychological Society,* **31**, 145–146.
Hersen, M., and Bellack, A. S. (eds) (1981). *Behavioral Assessment: A Practical Handbook*, 2nd ed. New York: Pergamon.
Horn, J. L. (1976). Human abilities: A review of research and theory in the early 1970s. *Annual Review of Psychology,* **27**, 437–485.
Kat, B. (1980). Working party on manpower planning: Exponential growth — but how long can it last? *Division of Clinical Psychology Newsletter,* **27**, 6–9.
Kent, G., and Clarke, P. (1981). Psychology and medical teaching. *Bulletin of The British Psychological Society,* **34**, 174–175.
Liddell, A., and Boyle, M. (1980). Characteristics of applicants to the M.Sc. in clinical psychology at the North East London Polytechnic. *Division of Clinical Psychology Newsletter,* **30**, 20–25.
Meltzoff, J., and Kornreich, M. (1970). *Research in Psychotherapy.* New York: Atherton.
Pond, A. (1978). In defence of eclecticism: A clinical psychologist's view of psychological theories. *Bulletin of The British Psychological Society*, **31**, 360–361.
Price, R.H. (1978). *Abnormal Behavior: Perspective in Conflict*, 2nd ed. New York: Holt, Rinehart & Winston.
Shapiro, M. B. (1975). The requirements and implications of a systematic science of psychopathology, *Bulletin of The British Psychological Society,* **28**, 149–155.
Smail, D. J. (1973). Clinical psychology and the medical model. *Bulletin of The British Psychological Society,* **26**, 211–214.
Trethowan, W. H. (1977). *The Role of Psychologists in the Health Services: Report of the Sub-Committee.* London: HMSO.
Vingoe, F. J. (1981). *Clinical Psychology and Medicine: An Interdisciplinary Approach*. Oxford: Oxford University Press.
Watts, F. N. (1980). The legal registration of psychologists: Some questions and answers. *Bulletin of The British Psychological Society,* **33**, 77–79.

Weiss, D., and Davison, M. L. (1981). Measurement of psychometrics. *Annual Review of Psychology,* **32**, 629–658.
White, J. G. (1972). What is wrong with clinical psychology? *Bulletin of The British Psychological Society,* **25**, 101–106.
Whitehead, A. (1978). The clinical psychologist — an applied scientist? *Bulletin of The British Psychological Society,* **31**, 224–226.
Williams, J. M. G. (1981). Postgraduate dissertations in clinical psychology 1977–1979. *Bulletin of The British Psychological Society,* **34**, 176–177.

The Practice of Clinical Psychology in Great Britain
Edited by A. Liddell


*Chapter 3*

# *Professional responsibility*

*Lionel R. C. Haward*

## INTRODUCTION

The responsibilities which clinical psychologists carry in professional life form an ever-changing and complex pattern of relationships between themselves and individuals and organizations to whom or for whom they are responsible. These relationships change as the organizational structures (clinics, institutions, the National Health Services, etc.) change. More subtle, but often more important, changes come from the changing attitudes of society. The clinical psychologist today is subject to political and ethical sensitivities undreamed of when the present writer entered the profession thirty years ago. Moreover, constraints and responsibilities come not only from social mores but from legislation as well. Thus any discussion on professional responsibility must be not only temporally limited but geographically as well, because each country has its own social customs, mores and laws, its own professional regulating bodies, and its own character of interprofessional relationships.

### Types of Responsibility

If professional responsibility is to be examined critically, it requires the simplifying of the complexities into some form of classification, examining each category of responsibility in isolation, and finally effecting some kind of synthesis by which the detailed knowledge thus acquired can be integrated to provide an overall picture of the responsibility network in the here and now situation.

There are several ways in which this can be done. The British Psychological Society (1974) classifies the responsibilities of the clinical psychologist according to the particular role being practised at the time, namely, clinician, scientist, and teacher.

An alternative method would be to look at the people for whom and to whom the clinical psychologist is responsible. In the simplest model, appropriate to a probationary grade of clinical psychologist, this may be limited to the patient on the one hand and to the Head of Department or clinical supervisor on the other. In most cases, this is too simple a model, even for the student clinician. In token economy projects, for example, the responsibilities may extend to many patients rather than just one, and to a wide range of members of other professions, such as nurses, occupational therapists, and so on, whose own professional status and responsibilities may in some cases be above, in other cases below, that of the clinical psychologist. A more realistic model would need to consider all the professional relationships which exist in the clinical practice of the psychologist, including those which exist within the Health Service structure as well as those without it. Responsibilities may exist, according to the precise nature of the psychologist's work with the patient, towards the parents, siblings, children or other relations of the parent, sometimes to the patient's visitors or those who accompany the patient to the psychology department. Members of other caring professions may come within the psychologist's line of responsibility, especially when they are the source of referral or will be supervising the patient when the psychologist has discharged his immediate duty to him or her. It may include other individuals formerly having some responsibility for the patient, such as prison medical officers, prison psychologists, and probation officers, or their equivalents in the Education Service, the SMO, educational psychologist, and teacher. It may also include hospital voluntary workers, members of the public visiting the psychology department on an 'open-day', and a vast population of strangers who, in the eyes of the law, are the clinical psychologist's 'neighbours' and to whom he owes a duty of care.

To use such a model of responsibility would require not a chapter but a whole book. Moreover, it would involve considerable redundancy of material, since each line of responsibility overlaps with others, and many persons to whom the clinical psychologist relates professionally share similar responsibilities.

## Medical Responsibility

The clinical psychologist, in his professional practice, comes closer to the role of the psychiatrist than to any other health worker, and this has led some psychologists to recommend that their profession should follow the medical model of responsibility. Hunt (1956) for example, says that psychology should adopt the basic responsibility of medicine in the field of illness and develop its own contribution within a collaborative framework. In practice this is just not feasible, for the medical practitioner is granted, or has imposed upon him, a wide range of professional responsibilities, by numerous statutes such as the National Health Service Act, the Mental Health Act, the Dangerous Drugs Act, and many more. In contradistinction, the clinical psychologist has no specific responsibilities designated by Parliament, neither does he carry the kind of professional responsibilities discussed so clearly in Cobb (1979) whose neglect can lead to legal sanctions.

**Legal, Ethical, and Moral Responsibilities**

One practical way of examining the professional responsibilities of the clinical psychologist is to separate them into three classes; (a) those that are enforceable in and by law, which will be referred to here as legal responsibilities; (b) those which are not enforceable by law but which have some practical sanctions attached to them enforceable by the psychologists' governing body. In the UK this body is the British Psychological Society, in the USA it will be the American Psychological Association; (c) those responsibilities for which persuasive power alone exists for their acceptance. Such a classification inevitably leads to an overlap of professional responsibilities, some of which will be adhered to by right-thinking clinicians regardless of sanctions, but which at the same time have been made explicit in a professional code of ethics enforceable by the psychologists' professional governing body, and are also embodied in common and/or statute law. A psychologist whose actions harm a patient, for example, has failed in his professional responsibility to the patient in all three ways — moral, ethical, and legal, and if such a consequence arises from professional negligence, which Americans call malpraxis, he may well have to suffer the consequences in his conscience, in being forced to leave his professional association, and in damages awarded against him for tort and possibly breach of contract. As a tortfeasor he may also suffer the further consequences of being asked to resign from his appointment, which, in the case of a National Health Service appointment, may be the end of his clinical career. Improper relations with a patient of the opposite sex will similarly be an abrogation of responsibility in all three areas, and can lead to similar consequences. Indeed, such conduct — or misconduct — can lead to additional sanctions under the criminal law by infringing the appropriate sections of both the Mental Health Act 1959 and the Sexual Offences Act 1956 and bring the offending psychologist to prison.

## LEGAL RESPONSIBILITIES

It will be obvious from the foregoing that legal responsibilities arise in both civil and criminal law. The three areas of law from which professional responsibilities arise are tort, breach of contract, and criminal law, and these will be considered separately below. Of these three areas, the law of tort is the most important, being the most pervasive of professional practice, the Lorelei rocks which has shipwrecked many a clinical mariner, and which has become so much a professional hazard that only the most temerous and shortsighted clinician would dare to practise without the assurance of adequate professional indemnity cover, provided either by his employer or by an independent insurance company. Because of its direct relevance to modern practice in clinical practice, and the vulnerability of the clinician to an increasingly litigious public, most of this chapter will be concerned with professional responsibility in respect of tortious liability. The other types of legal responsibility, namely the adherence to professional contracts and the avoidance of professional crimes, will be discussed briefly, together with the remaining two areas of professional responsibility, namely, ethical and moral.

## Professional Responsibility in Tort

Tort, from Norman French *tort* meaning 'wrong' is defined as a civil wrong for which the remedy is a common law action for unliquidated damages. By civil is meant that the wrong is redressable by private action which affects only the wrongdoer, or tortfeasor, and the person wronged; however, some torts, such as assault, are also crimes, because they affect the public by involving the police. It follows that no action follows a tort unless the aggrieved persons decide to initiate litigation. In doing so they become 'plaintiffs'. The wrong must be one which is recognizable at common law, and the essence of the tort is that the plaintiff's feelings have been hurt and he feels sufficiently grieved to seek and require redress. This is why the damages which may be awarded are 'unliquidated'. Unlike accident insurance which guarantees specific payment for specific injuries — loss of limb, loss of sight, etc., the Court has to take into account how aggrieved the plaintiff has reason to be. While his actual physical or financial loss may be taken into account, this is not the prime factor in fixing damages. Thus a psychologist can commit a tort without causing any tangible damage, for example seeing a private patient in his own time on hospital premises, known legally as *injuria sine damnum*. Conversely, a plaintiff may be financially damaged yet possess no legal redress, that is *damnum sine injuria*, such as having a rival private practice set up next door. As a common law offence, tort has no statutes or codified law to define and clarify the issues, each case being based entirely upon precedent. Since doctors have been sued since early times and clinical psychologists are late comers to the legal scene, it follows that any action in tort brought against them is likely to be based upon a medical parallel.

## The Litigious Society

It should be noted that litigation is increasing rapidly and the risk of being sued is many times greater today than it was only a decade ago. The medical profession is the most sued of all the professions, and the General Medical Council deal with over 600 complaints annually against general practitioners alone, while hospital doctors are the ones most frequently taken to Court. (In California, one physician in every four has been sued.) The contemporary role of the clinical psychologist in therapy brings the profession increasingly closer to psychiatry in terms of litigation risk, and every practising clinician needs to know how to avoid risk of litigation, and how to protect and defend himself should legal action be taken against him. Various reasons have been put forward for the rapid increase in litigation, and most of them operate in combination. They include the existence of Legal Aid, which is now available for civil action, although formerly restricted to defence against criminal charges. Potential litigants can now sue with nothing to lose and everything to gain by doing so, a situation which inevitably encourages litigation. Another factor is that more of the general public have a smattering of law, both through self-help books, such as *Family Lawyer*, and formal education in WEA and University Extension classes, at school — in 'A' Level Law, for example, and as part of a professional training in sociology, business studies, accountancy, and membership qualifications for professional institutions. Another factor is the greater understanding of the concept of 'rights' both through press articles and television programmes, government information leaflets, and the services of the Citizens' Advice Bureaux. There is, too, the fact of changing moral standards, with greed often transcending charitable attitudes, as for example when a mechanic was decapitated by an aircraft propeller and his grief-stricken widow was promptly sued by the owner for over £5,000 for damage to the propeller. Additionally, there is a long-standing attitude that faceless corporations and the Government are 'fair game' for which a different level of moral standard applies compared with that operating at interpersonal level, so that the disgruntled patient may well take action against a clinical psychologist knowing his employer, the NHS will pay the damages, but might hesitate to do so in private practice. An introduction to torts by psychologists has been given by Krauskopf (1965), and there are a number of especially relevant chapters in Schwitzgebel (1980), but any legal textbook on tort will provide a comprehensive understanding of the legal issues involved and the potentiality for committing tort in the practice of clinical psychology. The main divisions of tort of relevance to the practising clinician are those of trespass, defamation, and negligence, and these will be considered separately in some detail. Although trespass is generally associated with trespassing on private land (from its original Latin meaning *trans, pass* 'to go beyond' private boundaries), the legal meaning comes from the broader definition of transgression and is more akin to its use by Cranmer in the 1662 *Book of Common Prayer*; in the Lord's Prayer, for example, the supplicant prays to be forgiven his trespasses.

### *(i) Responsibility for trespass*

Legally, there are a variety of recognizable trespasses, which for convenience are classified into three groups, namely (i) trespasses against the person, (ii) trespasses against land, that is, real property or realty, and (iii) trespasses against property other than land, that is, personal property or personalty. It is worth repeating that the essence of the offence of tort is that the person so offended is aggrieved by having his rights unlawfully infringed. The actual consequences may be relevant to the damages awarded but not to the primary question of whether an offence has been committed. For the same reason, the *intention* of the tortfeasor is immaterial, unlike the general principle in criminal law where, the presence of *mens rea*, or criminal intent, is normally an essential element of the crime. The mental element in tort is therefore generally of no consequence, although there are certain exceptions where malice is an ingredient of the tort. If a psychologist acts maliciously against a patient, in the way he words the report, for example, he may be committing a tort where otherwise no offence would lie. Furthermore, the presence of malice may negate some recognized defence which the psychologist could otherwise raise to protect himself against the suit.

*Assault.* Although in popular language assault is construed as a physical attack, in law it has a restricted definition which was accorded it in the Middle Ages and still remains valid. An assault, legally, may be any act which arouses apprehension of hurt in the victim. It is defined as any act, short of physical contact, which a reasonable man could construe as threatening harm. Glanville Williams (1978) describes it as 'threatened battery', since it comes from the Latin *ad saltare* — 'to jump at'. Lord Goddard (1952), a Chief Justice, ruled in the case of Rolfe that 'an assault can be committed without touching a person'. The essence of the assault is the expectation of hurt. As Williams (*op. cit.*) states: 'The victim must expect that force is about to be applied to him. He need not experience fear, provided that he has that expectation.' In behaviour therapy, the tort of assault can be inadvertently committed by the clinical psychologist by the production of, for example, a vaginal dilator in treating vaginismus, or of an injector gun for carrying out a Funkenstein Test. Many people are nervous of electricity, and being brought into the presence of a polygraph or feedback apparatus may constitute a tort. Clearly the responsibility of the psychologist here lies in the adequate preparation of patients before confronting them with a situation which appears to be threatening in some way. Having suitably informed, reassured, and obtained the consent of the patient, the psychologist is better placed to defend himself against an aggrieved and litigious patient. Note that normally some action on the part of the psychologist is required to constitute the tort of assault, such as going towards the patient with the dilator or hypodermic syringe in his hand, or holding out the electrodes. Words alone are not usually enough to constitute assault, but action accompanied by the words ('I'm just going to insert this instrument') or a particular environment or milieu such as the presence of an instrument accompanied by words (e.g. 'This box gives shocks') could be regarded as assault. If, however, the words alone *cause* hurt to the patient, that is beyond the fear or expectation of hurt they become a tort in their own right. In the case of *Wilkinson* v. *Downton* (1897) the defendant as a joke told the plaintiff that her husband had had an accident, as a result of which the plaintiff suffered a nervous shock, and the Court ruled that a tort had been committed. Generally, the courts construe the tortious actions of professional workers in cases of assault as due to lack of care or thought rather than as deliberate conduct, and it is therefore more usual to sue for negligence rather than assault. Common assault is a crime as well as a tort, and at a recent general court martial, Deedes (1979), an officer, was charged with assault for firing a rifle at a recruit who did not realize it was loaded with blank ammunition, thus putting him 'in fear and apprehension'.

*Battery*. Battery is defined as touching a person against his will. Although associated with physical harm — battered babies and battered wives, for example, as a tort the offence is an affront to the person's dignity. This is why heavy damages are awarded for wrongful fingerprinting, which is also battery. Battery, like assault, is both a crime and a tort, although as a crime it must be some form of physical attack. The phrase 'assault and battery' used in criminal indictments indicates that the one is normally preceded by the other. Unlike assault, the patient when touched need not fear being hurt or harmed, but may merely be affronted. Thus the psychologist who puts a comforting arm round the shoulders of a distressed patient may inadvertently commit battery. Behaviour therapy is of course rife with potential batteries — injections, blood sampling for eosinophil counting, sphygmomanometry in treating hypertension, applying electrodes to monitor skin temperature, vasodilation, muscle tension, GSR and the like, inserting dental rolls in the mouth for the SHP Test or dilators in the vagina, or even carrying out the preliminary physical examination for BT are all potentially tortious procedures. Even brushing past a person has been declared by the Court to be tortious, as in *McGee* v. *Vanover* (1912).

*Mayhem*. If battery is a mere touch, what can one call a full-blooded attack of physical injury? Technically speaking, this is mayhem, which originally referred to any act which impairs the fighting qualities of the plaintiff, such as injury to a limb or loss of an eye. Body wounds not severe enough to stop him continuing the battle were excluded. Gradually the connotation was enlarged to include any serious consequences of battery, and the term is now becoming legally obsolete and exists mainly in literature where, like assault and battery, its original meaning has been greatly augmented and exaggerated. Mayhem is an unlikely tort for a clinical psychologist to commit, although one practitioner nearly became a defendant to a mayhem suit when the mental patient he was helping out of the psychology department tripped and fell down the stairs and accused him of having nudged her. In such simple ways the psychologist may become liable in law to damages accounting for many years' salary, and such examples highlight the need for professional indemnity insurance and a good personal relationship with the patient. Because of the adverse potentialities of behaviour therapy in trespass to the person, the legal problems involved have already reached the American Courts, although at the time of writing all instances involving psychologists in the United Kingdom are believed to have been settled out of Court. In the USA, in a long and complicated series of hearings extending over two years, *Wyatt* v. *Stickney* (1971–1973), certain standards of therapeutic care associated with behaviour therapy were laid down, and these have become accepted by many ethical committees as basic rules governing the use of behavioural therapies. The legal rules laid down in the Wyatt–Stickney case not only specify when and under what conditions certain types of treatment can be used, but specify precisely the qualifications and limitations attached to particular types of noci. For example Standard

XXIV(a) stipulates aversion therapy must be authorized by the hospital ethical committee as well as having the patient's consent, while XXIV(b) refers specifically to electric shocks, which are prohibited except for treatment of self mutilation, and then only if *all* available alternative therapies have been tried and failed. Where such standards are in force, or adopted as guidelines by the psychologists' professional bodies, the psychologist clearly has a responsibility to conform to them. His professional conduct, when tortious conduct is in issue, will always be assayed by the Court against the conduct of his peers, and any ethical code or rules of procedure adopted by them will be the standards against which the defendant psychologist will be judged.

*Innominate torts.* A fourth form of trespass against the person is one that falls uneasily between the other three. It occurs when the patient suffers some real injury — albeit psychological, such as a severely disabling neurotic reaction — although being neither touched by the therapist nor put in fear or expectancy of harm. The joke which misfired, mentioned earlier, is one example of what has become known as an innominate tort. A number of more professional examples sprinkle the annual reports of the Medical Defence Union and concern the conduct of psychiatrists, although the situations described could equally well apply to those encountered in clinical psychology. A typical case is reported in *Landau* v. *Werner* (1961), where a psychiatrist was held responsible by the Court for the *emotional damage* sustained by the patient as a result of the social contact she had previously enjoyed. All the cases on record have three elements in common: (1) the therapist is of the opposite sex to the patient; (2) the therapy involves social interaction between the therapist and the patient — for example, taking a phobic patient into a restaurant; and (3) the patient becomes aggrieved and 'affronted' when this part of the therapy is terminated. With emotionally unstable patients whose lives have been socially impoverished, the pleasures of a new social life with a high status and possibly young and attractive escort are often highly addictive, and withdrawal symptoms produced by too abrupt a termination of such a positively reinforcing procedure may be sufficient to produce a relapse or precipitate some more dramatic condition than the original one.

An added danger in this type of therapy is the possibility of 'countertransference', if one dare use an analytic concept in a behavioural context. Psychologists are only human, and have their weaknesses like everyone else (though they are expected to have more insight than others into their own weaknesses) and in the absence of a satisfying heterosexual relationship may find themselves especially vulnerable to an insidiously developing emotional attachment to a patient who happens to possess the appropriate qualities they need. The risks are the same for either sex, and at least one female psychologist has been successfully sued in Court by the patient's wife for what the Judge described as 'predatory psychotherapy'. The fact that the psychologist eventually married her patient was deemed to aggravate rather than mitigate the offence (*Savader* v. *Karp* (1978) ).

The misuse of a therapeutic relationship to develop sexual intimacy can become more a serious tort and of course overlaps the common law crime and a statutory offence under the Sexual Offences Act and Mental Health Act, etc. Such cases gain much publicity when brought before the General Medical Council. Medical practitioners risk losing their professional livelihood for such torts, as do clinical psychologists, for more than one clinician has found himself unable to secure professional employment after a forced resignation from the NHS. Less severe, but equally crippling financially, are the consequences following the innominate tort caused by telling the patient the diagnosis. A number of cases are on record where the patient has learnt that he or she is schizophrenic, and reacted with some adverse medical condition. In *Schneider* v. *Eisovitch* (1960) for example, information conveyed by a nurse to a patient produced a nervous shock which resulted in recurrent neurodermatitis, for which the patient recovered damages. It is natural for the psychologist to discuss the patient's condition and since he has access to the medical case-notes, there is always the possibility that he may let slip information which the consultant in charge had held back but which the psychologist had not realized was confidential to the patient. Since psychologists are often asked to carry out diagnostic tests, it is especially important for the profession to have an agreed policy on what, if anything, can be told to the patient direct. In some cases the psychologist is better placed than others to take on the responsibility of informing the patient of his condition, but in doing so the legal risks of committing an innominate tort must also be appreciated.

At the present moment the profession is exercised by the potential problems of the innominate tort inherent in certain clinical practices; these include hypnotic suggestion, implosion or flooding therapy using verbal stimuli; taped suggestions, and similar verbal inputs which are calculated to affect the patient.

*False imprisonment.* The final trespass against a person concerns any constraints upon the freedom of the patient. The patient need not even know at the time that his freedom has been constrained as in *Meering* v. *Graham White Aviation Co.* (1919) — e.g. keeping a patient waiting for a nurse escort, but knowledge of constraint increases the damages. False imprisonment can actually take place in the open with no physical barriers to the patient's escape, if the intention is not to allow the patient full freedom of movement, as in certain desensitization programmes. Some 'time-out' procedures are technically instances of unlawful imprisonment, and the Wyatt–Stickney Rules cover these situations explicitly. On one occasion a patient used the toilet of the psychology department when the psychologist in charge thought he had returned to the ward. He locked up and went home, leaving the patient imprisoned in the isolated hospital building. This is a typical situation leading to a suit for false imprisonment, although when the tortfeasor is a professional the solicitors acting for the plaintiff prefer to sue on negligence since they can recover greater damages that way. Fortunately for the psychologist this particular patient was too mentally disturbed to be aware of his rights. In the present climate of concern over patient care it would be more likely to promote an official enquiry and possible legal action brought by one of the patients' protection societies.

*Trespass to land.* Interference with possession of land is a tort, but, unlike trespass to the person, is not a crime. It includes entry on to land — the most usual meaning of 'trespass' in everyday speech, as well as remaining on land after permission to be there expires. It also includes entry on land for a purpose other than that for which permission has been granted, and also putting articles on land other than that owned by oneself.

It is important to realize that the clinical psychologist has no automatic right to go where he pleases in the institution in which he works, although permission to go where his *duty* may take him is implied. However, he may commit trespass by entering certain wards or non-medical buildings of the hospital without specific permission; or by leaving his personal possessions on hospital property (except his own quarters if he lives-in); or by entering the hospital for non-NHS business (seeing a private patient, for example). If his contract of employment is for specified hours of work, remaining late may be trespass. In the year 1610, the six carpenters' case introduced the concept of trespass *ab initio*, or trespass from the beginning. If a misfeasance, or offence by *active* conduct, is committed after lawful entry, the commission of the offence revokes the original authority to enter. Thus a psychologist committing a tort on hospital property, say trespass to the person, would be deemed to have committed trespass to land *ab initio* and could, in theory at least, be held liable for damages for this additional tort. In practice institutions do not concern themselves with trespass to land by their servants, but where complaints concerning unauthorized entry are made — often by a trade union representative in some status-dispute — the hospital authorites have been known to threaten action on the basis of this tort. One of the author's clinical students, whose presence on a certain ward was objected to by the nursing staff concerned, was threatened with legal action, and was transferred and eventually discharged from the course to avoid an escalation of consequences.

*Trespass to goods.* This tort is an interference with possession or ownership, the latter also being one of a number of different crimes, such as theft, conversion, etc. The psychologist, as a responsible professional worker, is expected to know and observe the difference between *meum* and *tuum*, but there has been a blurring of the ethical and moral distinctions in relation to employers of large and impersonal institutions, of which the Government is the largest. What traditionally is regarded as 'perks' may have no recognition in law, and when sample car checks and personal searches by the police are instituted at the request of a health authority after a spate of pilfering, the dispute over what property (stationery, books, apparatus) the psychologist may or may not be entitled to remove from the premises may be more than merely embarrassing to the psychologist concerned. Examination of some of the reports of hospital enquiries will reveal that not all psychologists have escaped unscathed from such investigations. It may not always be easy for the police to prove that the psychologist intended to permanently deprive the hospital of a stock of paper and envelopes; it is always more difficult for the psychologist to prove his possession of the articles was not tortious. This is an area where the legal, ethical, and moral responsibilities of clinical psychologists all coincide.

*(ii) Defamation*

One of the professional responsibilities of the psychologist is to convey information about the patient to a third party, who may be the patient's employer, family doctor, hospital consultant, or perhaps insurer. The competent and caring psychologist will want to be honest as well as diplomatic. However, it is not always possible to be both at one and the same time, and there will be occasions when what the psychologist has to say about the patient may be deeply offensive to him and prompt him to consider litigation. There are two kinds of defamation, namely slander, which is spoken and therefore transitory, and libel, which is written or in other respects permanent, and since it will continue to offend throughout the period of existence, is presumed to be more serious. Slander is a tort only, but libel is also a crime (in English law, but not in Scotland or the USA). The tort of defamation may be understood as a trespass against reputation: the justification for it being a crime is that by causing an injury to feelings it could lead to a breach of the peace. This makes it understandable why a tortious libel requires the involvement of three persons — the defamer, the defamed, and the third party to whom the defamed suffers a loss of reputation, whereas criminal libel requires only two persons to be involved. In tort, truth is a good defence, since the defamed then deserves his ill-reputation; however, in criminal libel truth is no defence except in certain cases; indeed, the rule is: 'the greater the truth, the greater the libel', because the defamed is more likely to be outraged by public revelation of the facts, and therefore more likely to breach the peace. Defamation is defined as any statement which falsely discredits, or exposes to hatred, ridicule or contempt, or causes the person identified to be shunned and avoided. Defamation is a common law offence but has been codified by various statutes from Fox's libel Act (1792) to the Defamation Act (1952).

*Slander.* The psychologist may commit slander unintentionally by dictating a letter about a patient, the secretary taking dictation becoming the necessary third party, or by telling a belligerent next-of-kin about the deficiencies of his or her relation. However, because of its transitory nature, slander is difficult to prove and an action for slander normally requires proof of damages sustained as a result of the slander, which are even more difficult to substantiate.

There are, however, four exceptions to the 'proof of damages rule' which increase the vulnerability of the clinical psychologist. These are (1) imputation of a criminal offence punishable by more than a fine, and of course many patients seen by the psychologist have criminal records which may be specially relevant to the purpose of his report on dangerousness in a Mental Health Review Tribunal for instance; (2) imputation of an existing contagious disease, now generally extended to infectious diseases and so making reports on venereal disease in sex clinic attenders open to this risk; (3) imputation of unchastity in a woman: adultery is stipulated in both common law and statute law (the Slander of Women Act, 1891) and lesbianism entered case law with Keer and Kennedy 1941, both circumstances which figure prominently in sex therapist's reports; and (4) words calculated to disparage in office, profession, calling, trade or business. Thus in *Howe* v. *Prinn* (1702) it was held not actionable to call a magistrate 'an ass and a beetle-headed justice': the Bench got its own back nearly 300 years later (Peterborough, 1980) when the Court of Appeal ruled that the magistrate who called the accused 'a clown, an idiot, a ratbag, a nit, a clot, and a dickhead' was merely expressing an opinion!

*Libel.* Although most libellous statements are written, and in medical cases occur in reports or letters to other doctors, the statement need not be verbal. A film depicting Rasputin raping the Russian Princess was held to be libel (*Youssoupoff* v. *M.G.M.*, 1934). An advertising cartoon showing a golf champion with a bar of Fry's chocolate sticking out of his pocket was regarded as libel (Tolley *v*. Fry, 1931). And when Tussauds created an wax effigy of a man they were having an altercation with, and put it among the murderers in their Chamber of Horrors, that was held to be libel, too (*Monson* v. *Tussauds*, 1894). Radio, TV broadcasts, and tape recording, are statutorily defined as libel although they would otherwise be regarded as slander. Libel does not require proof of damage but does require proof, in tort, that a third party saw it, that it actually was identified with the plaintiff, and that it was defamatory. For an action for defamation to succeed, the court requires evidence which will prove these facts, namely that the statement was defamatory, that it was published to a third party, and that it identified the plaintiff.

*Proof of defamation*. As we have seen in slander, vulgar abuse is not considered in law to be defamatory, and the jury seem to have no difficulty generally in differentiating the two. Thus when Westcote said: 'You blackguard, rascal, scoundrel; Penfield, you are a thief,' the jury ruled that the first three nouns were vulgar abuse but the fourth was defamatory (*Penfield* v. *Westcote*, 1806). Moral discredit is not necessary for defamation, and statements of innocent conditions such as being a rape victim, a mental patient, or intellectually subnormal have given rise to actions for defamation. Since the clinical psychologist spends much of his professional life making statements about the last two and at least occasionally about the first, there is obviously some need to be concerned about potential risks in this tort. Defamation is often implicit rather than explicit and may be mere innuendo, as in the chocolate-carrying golfer cartoon mentioned above. So, too, when the *Daily Mirror* announced in mistaken innocence that A and B had become engaged, they became guilty of defaming A who was already married to C, since it implied A and C were unmarried and therefore living in sin (*Cassidy* v. *Daily Mirror*, 1929). The judge is responsible in deciding in the first instance whether the statement is capable of being defamatory, that is whether there is a *prima facie* case. If there is, he permits the action to continue and after hearing all the evidence the jury decide whether the defamation has been satisfactorily proved. The test they applied is known as Lord Aitkens Test which can be summarized as: 'would the words tend to lower the plaintiff in the estimation of right-thinking members of society' (*Sin* v. *Stretch*, 1936).

*Proof of publication*. Although only two parties are necessary in criminal libel, publication to a third party must be proved in tort. The spouse of the defamer is not considered a third party in these circumstances, because for many centuries husband and wife were regarded in English law as only one person, and the separation is still not complete. However, the spouse of the defamer is, because a person may be most humiliated in front of the spouse than before any number of less intimate people. 'Open' correspondence, such as postcards, telegrams, dictated correspondence, etc., are legally recognized as forms of publication, as are letters to third parties unless rebutted, but where the third party wrongfully obtains access to a letter, as when the butler opens one's letter (*Huth* v. *Huth*, 1915) publication is rejected. 'Innocent disseminators' are not liable, but newsagents and booksellers are liable for posters (*Sunlife Assurance* v. *W. H. Smith*, 1933), and, of interest to psychologists, editors and authors are legally under a special duty to ascertain the nature of the text with which they are concerned.

*Proof of identity*. It is not necessary for the defamed to be actually identified by name — since as we have seen, a recognizable cartoon, film scene, or wax effigy has proved sufficient proof in past cases. Defamation runs against the defamer, so if a report on patient A also innocently identifies patient B of whom it is untrue, then B can take action against the psychologist, to whom he may be quite unknown. Thus when the Express Newspapers reported a bigamy case against Harold Newstead, a barman of Camberwell, a hairdresser of the same name recovered damages (*Newstead* v. *Express*, 1940).

Even an imaginary character can be identified with a real person to the liability of the creator, which is why authors and film producers make an explicit denial that their characters resemble any real person, living or dead. Even the most fortuitous sequence of imaginative events may be paralleled in real life, as Hultons found out, when they published a story about Artemeous Jones, an imaginary character described as an upright pillar of society but keeping a mistress in Dieppe. The print was hardly dry when a real Artemeous Jones stood up, declaring he was not only a pillar of society and a church warden to boot, but was also a barrister-at-law. That was a costly exercise of imagination for the author (*Jones* v. *Hulton*, 1910).

It should be noted from the above that once the requisite proof of defamation, publication, and identity is made, it is no excuse that the plaintiff was not the intended defamed person, or that the statement itself (which on one occasion was a simple statement of IQ) was not intended to be defamatory, or that the psychologist was only repeating what another person (his colleague, a nurse, the consultant) had said. Even explicitly qualifying a statement as a rumour does not remove the defamatory element; in *Watkin* v. *Hall* (1868) the statement: 'You have heard the rumour that the Chairman has failed' was held to be defamatory.

*Defences in defamation.* There are a number of different ways a psychologist sued for defamation can defend himself, by denial, pleas, apology and offer of amends. He may deny that the statement is defamatory, but unless he can convince both judge and jury this will not help. A clinician spends his life amongst psychiatric patients and may not regard their condition as defamatory, but as one juror said in a relevant case: 'a nutter is still a nutter' and mental abnormality is still in a social shadow and requires ever-changing euphemisms to become acceptable. The psychologist may deny publication, and this is a matter of fact or a matter of law, rather than a matter of opinion.

There are three pleas that can be made — truth, privilege, or fair comment of public interest.

*Truth as defence in defamation.* Truth is no defence in criminal libel, indeed truth is a weapon for the prosecution, for the rule is: 'the greater the truth, the greater the libel'. In tortious libel, however, justification is a good defence. It need not be true in every minor detail, but must be *substantially true*. This approximation gives the law some leeway: thus a court ruled that the statement that the plaintiff had been sent to prison for *three* weeks for travelling on the railway without a ticket was substantially true, even though it was proved he had been imprisoned for *two* weeks for the offence. In this case 'substantially true' was construed as 'two-thirds correct'.

On this basis the statement was justified. More recently, when the author of *Exodus* wrote that Dr Dering of North London had taken part in 17,000 experimental operations on prisoners in Auschwitz, it was proved that he had undertaken a substantial number of such operations, but not 17,000, and the statement in the book was therefore not legally justified. That the court thought it was *morally* justified was indicated by the award of ½d damages. To be accepted as a defence, the statement must be true at the time it was made. Referring to someone as a mental patient when they are no longer under treatment or care as such leaves the psychologist fully liable.

The justification may be based on opinion. Prokop (1974) is a psychologist who severely criticized a book on parapsychology. He was sued by the book's author, a man of many learned publications, but successfully defended his review on the grounds of justification, giving the court a clear exposition of the scientific basis for his criticisms. However, the likelihood of justification based on opinion succeeding will depend entirely upon whether the jury share the same opinion as the defamer. Prokop was lucky in that his jury favoured a materialistic explanation.

Reviews, which by their very nature call for criticisms, obviously carry a risk of legal liability to the psychologist reviewer, but even the writing of scientific articles can be a risky business in the law of defamation. The longest libel trial in history concerned a member of the BMA who sued the authors of a research article on the grounds that they implied dishonesty of data interpretation. It was obviously a case whose solution rested upon the technicalities of research methodology and modern statistical analysis, and long before the issues could be resolved by the court, the litigants had argued themselves close to bankruptcy. The case was eventually settled out of court.

In another case of special relevance to psychologists the plaintiff was also swimming against the tide of jury opinion. In this case, the scientist was called to give expert evidence in a case brought under the Race Relations Act 1965. Commenting upon the case, the *Sunday Times* said that the defence had called 'Expert' evidence which was interpreted as having proposed the congenital superiority of the white race. The ethnologist sued the paper for libel on the grounds that the use of quotation marks implied he was not an expert and that the comment implied he was a racialist. The *Sunday Times* called in distinguished experts who put forward a contrary argument to that of the ethnologist, and the plaintiff lost to a majority verdict.

*Plea of privilege.* A second plea in defence of defamation is that of privileged communication, and this is the defence most commonly used by psychologists and other members of the health professions. Some statements have absolute privilege, such as anything said in Parliament, which is protected by the Bill of Rights (1689), or reported from Parliament (Parliamentary Papers Act 1840). Court proceedings have absolute protection, however false or malicious the statements may be, and this includes law reports and also communications between lawyers and clients.

Psychologists, like medical practitioners and other professionals are not granted absolute privilege, but they can claim qualified privilege in those instances where they have a legal, social, or moral duty to communicate to a recipient who has a corresponding interest to receive it (per Lord Justice Atkinson in *Adams* v. *Ward* (1917) ).

In order to use qualified privilege as a defence the psychologist must prove that his statement fell into one of the following four categories; namely, (1) discharge of duty: for example giving testimonials, providing reports to referring doctors, providing annual assessment on subordinate staff or students; (2) protecting interests, such as warning of a dishonest staff member; (3) reports in the public interest made to authority — as when psychologists in one hospital department made libellous complaints about their Head of Department to NHS Administrators and the British Psychological Society; and (4) fair and accurate reports of official proceedings, such as those of mental health review tribunals, for which psychologists frequently provide evidence. These tribunals enjoyed absolute privilege under common law but have been explicitly limited to qualified privilege by the Defamation Act (1952).

Additionally, in claiming qualified privilege, psychologists must comply with certain conditions, such as having good faith (showing no malice, spite, or ill will and taking care to ascertain the truth of the matter), limiting the statement to scope of duty and purpose, and making them in a proper manner and on a proper occasion. A psychologist who in a formal report states that a patient is schizophrenic may be protected by qualified privilege. If he is overheard telling the referring doctor this at the staff party (because he feels the matter is urgent) he has forfeited his claim to this defence. Thus in *Iverson* v. *Frandsen* (1956) the Court decided that the report by a psychologist to a referring psychologist which stated that the plaintiff was 'feeble minded on the Stanford-Binet' was qualified privilege, whereas a report that an employee was 'psychologically unreliable for detailed responsibility' was considered defamatory on the grounds that, although true, made properly and as part of the examiner's duty, it was not made in good faith, and cost the defendant nearly a year's salary, *Chaudhary* v. *Cowan* (1973). In *Berry* v. *Monch* (1958) a general practitioner asked a therapist for the diagnosis of a particular patient, as the parents of the girl to whom he had become engaged, were concerned about his desirability as a future son-in-law. The therapist replied that the patient was a psychopath, that he left the hospital owing money, and that the girl should run away from him as fast as she could. The patient got to hear of this letter in the altercations which followed and sued his therapist, who claimed qualified privilege the letter being written from one health professional to another on a medical matter. The court queried whether any of the conditions had been met for this defence. The GP had no professional connection with the patient, and the defendant therefore had no duty to report on his condition. The therapist did not take care to ascertain the truth of his statements, and wrote about his patient with ill will. Moreover, although asked for the diagnosis, he went beyond the enquiry and gratuitously gave his opinion on the prospects of the marriage. Clearly, since much of what clinical psychologists report is *prima facie* libellous in law, it behoves them to ensure that they enjoy the protection of qualified privilege, and this can only be done by knowing, understanding, and complying with all the rules.

*Defence of fair comment.* Fair comment of public interest is often used as a defence in cases of libel in scientific writings since the qualified privilege defence is not appropriate. Prokop (*op. cit.*) could have used it to defend his psychological review. Virtually all the cases involving scientific criticism have been settled out of court, which makes it difficult to assess the effectiveness of fair comment as a defence. The courts themselves are somewhat equivocal on this issue. In *Drummond-Jackson* v. *BMA* (1970) the plaintiff's method of using intravenous methahexone had been attacked. Lord Denning was of the opinion that this was lawful criticism, being both impersonal and objective, and therefore the defence of fair comment applied. Lord Salmon, however, took the contrary view, and regarded an attack on a therapeutic technique as an attack on the person associated with its discovery or introduction. In Lord Salmon's view, to say of a practitioner he uses a bad technique is to say he is a bad practitioner, and thus cannot be fair comment. Psychologists with modest savings would therefore do well to examine their critiques of fellow professionals carefully before publishing them.

*Statutory apology.* This defence was introduced by the Libel Act (1843) generally known as Lord Campbell's Act, and refers only to libels published in periodicals. The defendant pleads that the libel was made without malice or gross negligence, publishes a full apology at the earliest opportunity in the same periodical, and pays compensation into court. This defence is not popular since no other defence is permitted and it is virtually a plea of guilty which leaves the defendant vulnerable to both the court and the aggrieved party.

*Offer of amends.* Lord Campbell's statutory apology has been brought up to date by Section 4 of the Defamation Act 1952. The defendant must show that he published the libel innocently and without malice, used reasonable care to ascertain the truth, did not know the words were defamatory or did not know they could be applied to the plaintiff and published an apology and correction to all who may have received the libellous matter. If the offer is accepted, the action is closed and the court orders costs and expenses, which in the absence of dispute will be relatively small. If the offer is rejected, the offer itself is a defence and the court takes this into consideration when judging the issue and awarding damages and expenses. It is important to appreciate that the litigant winning the case may enjoy a moral victory but may lose more in reputation and real money than the litigant who loses. Thus Dr Dering won his action against Leon Uris but received only ½*d* compensation and had to pay his own and most of the defendant's costs, a sum approaching £100,000.

### *(iii) Negligence*

Negligence has emerged as a tort in its own right, although it may be an essential ingredient of other torts, such as trespass or defamation, and occurs in other non-tortious civil offences like breach of contract. In criminal law negligence appears as criminal negligence, and the psychologist may be found guilty of this crime if the patient suffers severely as a result. Criminal prosecutions for negligence in the NHS are comparatively infrequent, perhaps because of the difficulty of finding fellow-professionals willing to testify against one of their own kind and the last case reported was in 1974. Psychologists in charge of departments, or of subordinate psychologists, have had a further responsibility imposed since 1975, when the Health and Safety at Work Act was introduced. Under this statute a breach of duty in negligence may become a breach of statutory duty; thus a tort is converted to a crime, and the psychologist found against can face two years imprisonment and an unlimited fine.

Professional negligence in English law emerged in 1534 AD and surgeons become liable during the Wars of the Roses. In 1932 the famous 'snail in the bottle' case opened up the duty of care to extend to all who might be at risk by foreseeable consequences. Medical negligence, which pertains to the clinical practice of psychologists, requires and indeed possesses a book to itself (Nathan and Barrowclough, 1957) and the reader should refer to this text and such articles as Knight (1976). Since most actions for torts against psychologists will either include the notion, or be on the basis, of negligence, responsibility for good professional practice is of first importance to the clinical psychologist. The standard of care he is expected to exercise is that appropriate to his professional peers in the same NHS grade. Senior psychologists naturally shoulder responsibility for juniors, and if the latter are sued for negligence, the supervising senior, whether present at the time or not, can expect to be joined in the suit as a joint tortfeasor. The standards of care are judged in court by calling other members of the profession to testify as to their own practice, and it is against this criterion, rather than any unrealistic ideal, that the psychologist will be judged.

According to the Medical Defence Union (1971), detailed and accurate notes are a necessity if any defence is to succeed, since rebuttal of negligence usually requires reference to contemporaneous notes. All writers on the subject stress the need for comprehensive records and while each psychologist carries the responsibility for recording all essential information on his interaction with the patient, the Head of Department or District Service has responsibility for the overall policies concerning psychology records.

### *(iv) General defences*

In an action for defamation, special defences were described which have developed by statute law. For all torts, however, there are certain general defences available which can be used as appropriate. As a general rule *mistake* is no defence, but it can be used in certain circumstances where malice is a necessary ingredient. *Inevitable accident* is another defence, but not always easy to maintain, since it requires proof that the defendant took *all* the precautions a reasonable man would take. The effectiveness of 'working to rule' as a method of interfering with everyday work routines is evidence enough that the accepted pace of professional life prevents the psychologist from being as meticulous as the court would expect. *Necessity* is a third defence, when a tort is committed to prevent a greater wrong; for example, locking up an actively suicidal patient until nursing help can be obtained or physically subduing an assaultive patient. *Statutory authority* is a defence against actions for torts committed as part of that duty. The psychologist employed by the NHS is empowered to treat a patient detained under Section 26 of the Mental Health Act against his will so that no action brought against the psychologist for battery by aversion therapy, say, would succeed as long as it was indicated in the view of the psychologist's professional peers, and that the psychologist had been given the responsibility for dealing with the patient by the responsible Medical Officer. Moves are afoot to protect the S26 patient from such infringement of rights, but legislation increasingly reduces private and personal rights for the alleged benefit of society. However, the most important defence for the clinician will always be the *consent* of the patient, known legally by the following Latin title.

*Volenti non fit injuria.* The principle is: 'He who consents cannot claim for injury' and an important part of professional practice is to obtain the written consent of the patient for any procedure from which some form of detrimental sequelae might follow. While the need for explicit consent is obvious in the use of aversion therapy, injections, blood sampling, and biofeedback, it will be remembered that innominate torts can arise out of mere words or innocent conduct, so that a good case can be made for obtaining the formal consent of the patient for all procedures offered, even simple counselling, and especially when the psychologist and patient are of opposite sex. The MDU (1974) has a small publication on consent, and Farndale (1975) enlarges on the legal aspects of consent forms. Consent need not be written or even explicit — a patient who holds out his arm to have electrodes taped on may be said to be implicitly consenting to the procedure. But as a defence against tortious liability, the law requires more than consent, it requires informed consent. The problems inherent in obtaining consent from the psychiatric patient have been well expressed by Gostin (1980) but they are perhaps more difficult in the case of mentally handicapped adults. One excellent method has been devised by the psychologists of the Hampshire Standing Committee on Mental Handicap, who have incorporated a simple questionnaire into the consent form, the completion of which is *prima facie* evidence of the patient's understanding of the treatment.

*Professional indemnity.* The clinical psychologist will normally be indemnified against litigation by the NHS under the same terms of the Mental Health Act as that enjoyed by nurses and other professional workers. However, this only applies to alleged torts committed as acts which are specifically and acceptably part of the contract of employment. With psychologists tending to work further and further away from medical supervision, their claim for support becomes correspondingly weaker, so that in one case where a behaviour therapist was brought before a court by an aggrieved patient, the consultant psychiatrist, far from authenticating the treatment, gave evidence that in his opinion the treatment was unnecessary. In these circumstances the need for individual insurance is manifest.

## ETHICAL RESPONSIBILITY

Most of this chapter has been taken up with the *legal* responsibilities of the psychologist, because these are of primary importance and also are the professional responsibilities which are most precisely defined. In contradistinction, ethical responsibilities, although based upon generally agreed principles, are still controversial in many areas. The comprehensive guide by Van Hoose and Kottler (1977) makes clear the differences between the ethical and legal issues facing the psychologists working in a medically defined setting, and Hunt (1956) has suggested that clinical psychology should accept 'the basic responsibility of medicine'. Because the professional duties of the psychologist are not recognized statutorily as are those of the medical profession, the responsibilities borne by the two professions are dissimilar and can never be identical. Moreover, even psychiatry has responsibilities of a substantially different nature to those of clinical psychology, as Cobb's recent series (1979) makes manifest, so that clinical psychology has to look elsewhere for its ethical code. The most complete summary of a code of professional ethics is probably that published by the American Psychological Association (1953). Although designed for qualified clinicians, Wallen (1956) points out that students are also expected to observe these Rules. In the USA, specialized branches of psychology have developed their own supernumerary codes of ethics, such as the ADAMHA guidelines developed by the US Department of Health and discussed by Shah and Leabman (1977). In America, too, as noted earlier in examining the behaviour therapists' legal responsibilities in tort, some of the relevant ethical rules governing the practice of therapy have been embodied into legal rules and become case law. In the UK the tendency has been to avoid specifying too closely the individual acts which would constitute a perceived infringement of accepted ethical principles, and to move instead towards general guidelines for the direction of professional conduct. The British Psychological Society, under the terms of its Royal Charter, has the responsibility of 'compelling' the observance of strict rules of professional conduct as a condition of membership. Since eligibility for graduate membership of the BPS is one of the conditions laid down by the Whitley Council for appointment as a clinical psychologist in the NHS it can be seen that the former professional body can apply the utmost sanction to Health Service psychologists. Standards of professional conduct were laid down by the BPS in 1955 and revised and published as guidelines for the professional practice of clinical psychologists in 1974 by the Clinical Division. Every clinical psychologist working in the UK should possess a copy.

## MORAL RESPONSIBILITY

The clinician plies his profession within the guidelines of the law and his professional ethics. The two are always complementary and never in opposition, for it is an accepted ethical principle that the professional worker should be a law-abiding citizen, and no professional body would promulgate ethical rules which ran counter to the law as it prevailed at the time. (Trade Unions and certain political parties take a rather different view.) However, each clinician has to live with his conscience, and from time to time his own moral standards may clash with those existing in law or professional ethics. Usually such clashes come from the age-old dilemma of choosing between the good of the individual or the good of society — for example, what does the psychologist do when his patient admits to rape — preserve his patient's confidence and confidentiality or protect his community? The individual circumstances and the nature of the psychologist concerned will determine the final decision, but sometimes moral scruples can only be satisfied by acting unlawfully or unethically. More than one psychologist has faced prison to protect his patient's interests. Sometimes the moral conflict concerns not an individual versus Society, but where the moral responsibility lies between two individuals, a situation frequently occurring in child custody cases where one of the parents is a psychiatric patient being treated by the psychologist. Such personal problems may be quite harrowing for the latter; their alleviation comes from frequent discussion of such legal, ethical, and moral issues and responsibilities between clinicians, so that experiences can be shared, decisions discussed and justified, and more unifying moral ideas developed and accepted.

## REFERENCES

*(Legal cases cited will be found in the law reports of the year quoted.)*

American Psychological Association (1953). *Ethical Standards of Psychologists.* Washington, D.C.: APA.

British Psychological Society (1974). *Current Guidelines for the Professional Practice of Clinical Psychologists.* Leicester: BPS.

Cobb, J. (1979). *Responsibility in Psychiatry, Parts I–IV*. Welwyn: Smith, Kline and French.

Deedes, J. (1979). *Daily Telegraph*, 12th September.

Farndale, W. A. J. (1975). *Law on Hospital Consent Forms.* Beckenham: Ravenswood.

Gostin, L. (1980). *In Hazardous and Irreversible Treatments in Psychiatry — Who Decides?* Welwyn: Smith, Kline and French.

Hunt, W. A. (1956). *Clinical Psychology*. Springfield: Thomas.

Knight, B. (1976). Forensic problems in practice: II Medical negligence. *Practitioner,* **216**, 213–217.

Krauskopf, J. M. and O. J. (1965). Torts and psychologists. *Journal of Counselling Psychology,* **12**, 227–237.

Medical Defence Union (1971). Case Notes are vital. *Medical News Tribune,* 11th October.

Medical Defence Union (1974). Consent to treatment. London: MDU.

Nathan, Lord and Barrowclough, A. R. (1957). *Medical Negligence.* London: Butterworth.

Peterborough (1980). Nothing Personal. *Daily Telegraph*, 6th October.

Prokop, O. (1974). Judgment in a case involving parapsychology. *Kriminalische und Forensische Wissenschaft,* **14**, 105–108.

Schwitzgebel, R. L., and R. K. (1980). *Law and Psychological Practice.* Chichester: Wiley.

Shah, S. A., and Leabman, A. K. (1977). ADAMHA guidelines for the protection of human subjects. *World Journal of Psychosynthesis,* **9**, 34–37.

Van Hoose, W. H., and Kottler, J. A. (1977). *Ethical and Legal Issues in Counselling and Psychotherapy.* London: Jossey-Bass.

Wallen, R. W. (1956). *Clinical Psychology*. London: McGraw-Hill.
Williams, G. L. (1978). *Textbook of Criminal Law*. London: Sweet and Maxwell.

The Practice of Clinical Psychology in Great Britain
Edited by A. Liddell


*Chapter 4*

# *Organization of psychological services*

*Frank M. McPherson*

This chapter is about how clinical psychology is organized in the National Health Service, and deals both with the organization of services, and with the internal management structure of clinical psychology departments.

## HISTORICAL INTRODUCTION

The changes which have occurred in the organization of clinical psychology in recent years have to a large extent reflected more general changes within the NHS.

### Clinical Psychology Services Prior to 1974

For the first three decades after its inception in 1948, the health services provided by the NHS were unsatisfactory in three main respects: (i) undue emphasis was placed on hospital, as opposed to community and preventive, services; (ii) there was little systematic planning of health care; and (iii) services were fragmented and uncoordinated, and subject to major local variations.

Similarly, most clinical psychologists were employed to provide a service to specific hospitals or units. Because of the traditional association with psychiatry, these were mainly mental illness and mental subnormality hospitals, and clinical psychologists consequently had little contact with other branches of medicine, or with the community. Secondly, and more important for the development of the profession, clinical psychologists had relatively little contact with one another. Within a single town or district, several clinical psychology departments might exist, administratively independent of one another, and often having few professional links. Thirdly, the distribution of posts within a locality usually depended more on historical accident, or the entrepreneurial skills of individuals, than on a systematic appraisal of the needs of the population. Thus, it frequently occurred that one hospital had several psychologists in post, whereas a neighbouring one, serving an identical population, had none. Management arrangements were equally unsatisfactory, and many clinical psychologists were administratively, and some were professionally, accountable to doctors such as physician superintendents and in some cases even individual consultants.

## The Reorganizations of the NHS

The major reorganization of the NHS which occurred in 1974 after a long period of consultation was intended to remedy these general deficiencies by creating organizational and managerial structures which would facilitate the comprehensive planning and provision of the whole range of health services for entire communities.

The following are those features of the reorganized NHS which were particularly relevant to clinical psychology.

### *Organization of NHS services*

After 1974, in England a three-tier structure existed of Regions, Areas and Districts at the head of which was the Secretary of State for Social Services, a Cabinet minister who acts through the Department of Health and Social Security (DHSS). The DHSS is responsible for national planning, and for allocating resources to the fourteen Regional Health Authorities (RHAs), which interpret these national plans according to local circumstances, provide some services, and which, until 1982, financed and monitored the work of the Area Health Authorities (AHAs). The ninety AHAs were the main operational planning units of the NHS, and each was responsible for assessing the health needs of its population of a half to one million, and for planning services to meet these needs. Regions and Areas were thus concerned primarily with planning, but day-to-day management and provision of clinical services was the responsibility of the Districts, into which Areas were divided.

After a period of some confusion and uncertainty, these arrangements appeared to work well in most parts of the country. However, ostensibly to save a quite small sum of money, the Government introduced another reorganization, which took effect in 1982. The Area tier was abolished, and 182 new District Health Authorities were set up, each of which combines the planning function previously undertaken by Area with the service provision role already undertaken by District. Districts are often based on the catchment area of a general hospital and are intended to be large enough to provide the full range of medical and related services, while being still sufficiently small to maintain a coherent identity. The average District contains 275,000 people.

The health services in Scotland and Wales are to a large extent administratively independent of the NHS in England, and — in particular in Scotland — some differences exist also in the policies which are introduced for service provision. However, the same conditions of service, professional standards, etc. exist in all three countries. Organizationally, the main difference is that there are no Regions in Scotland or Wales: Departments of the Scottish and

Welsh Offices combine some of the functions of the DHSS with some of those of RHAs. Beneath the central Departments, each country is divided into Areas (Health Boards in Scotland, AHAs in Wales) which have a major responsibility for the planning of services; each Area is usually divided into Districts, which undertake the management of services.

### *Management of NHS*

Since the 1982 reorganization, the legal responsibility for the provision of health services in each locality in England rests, under the Secretary of State, with the Regional Health Authorities (RHAs) and District Health Authorities (DHAs). Each Authority comprises twenty or so unpaid members who meet regularly under a part-time chairman, and who are appointed by the Secretary of State after consultation with local authorities, professional and voluntary bodies, the universities, etc. However, the execution of policies, and the management of services, is mainly the task of full-time, appointed officers at Regional and District level. Of particular importance are the four-person 'teams of officers' which exist at each tier, and comprise medical, nursing and lay administrators, and a finance officer. Each team is collectively responsible for the efficient implementation of the administrative and clinical policies agreed by their Authorities, and each member also has specific responsibilities. In addition to these 'teams', various other officers are appointed to be responsible for particular professions or services; there are Regional Works Officers, District Dental Officers, District Occupational Therapists, and so on. The District Management Teams, in addition to the four full-time officers, also contain two elected medical members, one representing hospital doctors and the other, family practitioners.

Arrangements in Scotland and Wales are roughly similar.

## The Trethowan Report

These general features of the NHS, as it existed after the 1974 reorganization, but prior to 1982, influenced the only major official statement to have been made about the organization and management of clinical psychology services, the Trethowan Report. The Zuckerman Report (1968) on the organization of hospital scientific services had considered, but could not decide, whether clinical psychology should be included in the proposed integrated scientific service. Because of this uncertainty, and because of the imminent reorganization of the NHS, the DHSS Standing Mental Health Advisory Committee formed a sub-committee in 1972 under Professor W. H. Trethowan 'to consider the role of psychologists in the health services'. The Report was published in 1977, and several of its thirty Recommendations concerned the organization and management of services.

The Secretary of State, in Health Circular HC (77) 14, appeared to accept the Report although, since its publication coincided with one of the regularly recurring periods of financial stringency in the NHS, he commended to

Authorities only those Recommendations which had no immediate financial implications. However, the Report was welcomed by the profession, through the British Psychological Society, and it has been widely accepted as providing an appropriate model for clinical psychology services. Much of the remainder of this chapter will therefore comprise an outline and evaluation of the Trethowan Report Recommendations.

## THE ORGANIZATION OF CLINICAL PSYCHOLOGY SERVICES

### Trethowan Recommendations

As noted above, prior to 1974 most clinical psychologists were employed by, and provided services to, particular hospitals. In line with the philosophy of the reorganized NHS, the Report on the other hand recommended that clinical psychology should provide an integrated service to a community.

#### *Area departments of clinical psychology*

Paragraph 5.3.2 of the Report recommended that services should be organized on an Area basis, and be provided by 'Area Departments of Clinical Psychology'. The Report did not discuss in detail what exactly it meant by the term 'Area Department', but it is clear from the general context that more was implied than a loose administrative arrangement for co-ordinating services. Three features appeared to be important.

(i) *Contractual features.* Where an Area Department existed, all NHS clinical psychologists employed in that Area would belong to this single Department, rather than be employed by individual hospitals or services. A clinical psychologist might be associated closely with a specific hospital, but his/her contract of employment and Job Description would make him/her accountable to the employing Authority through the Area Department rather than through that hospital.

(ii) *Terms of reference.* The terms of reference, or professional responsibilities, of an Area Department would be very different from those, for example, of a traditional hospital Department. Whereas the latter is concerned only with those clients who are referred to it, an Area Department would have a responsibility to the *entire population* of the Area. This does not mean that services would necessarily be spread thinly over the whole Area, or that individual psychologists would spend most of their time travelling from unit to unit. Indeed, the Department might decide that the most effective use of its resources would be to concentrate exclusively on a few specific hospitals or client groups. Rather, the implication was that, in allocating its resources, the Department would take account of the needs of the population as a whole, and not merely those of a particular unit or service. The question which an Area

Department would ask itself was: 'How can existing resources be deployed so that they can most effectively prevent and reduce psychological distress and disorder in the entire Area?'.

(iii) *Administrative features.* In order that it might use its resources in ways in which it considers would maximize its effectiveness, an Area Department would have a considerable degree of administrative autonomy. One aspect of this — the contracts of individual members — has already been referred to. Another particularly important requirement is that the Department should have a large measure of control over its budgets, that is the money made available by the employing Authority for payment of psychologists' salaries, and travelling expenses, and for the purchase of supplies and equipment. Thus, for example, the Department should have the major say in determining how the staffing budget should be allocated. Of course, in these and other similar decisions, the Department would work within the constraints imposed by the resources available, and would take account both of the general policies of the Authority, and of the advice of other, related professions.

Three points should be made about this Recommendation. First, the choice of Area as the unit of organization reflected the low numbers of clinical psychologists. The District would have been a more logical choice since the Area dealt mainly with planning and it was the District which was concerned with service provision. The Report did indeed consider whether, to fit into the general pattern of health services, clinical psychology also ought to have been organized on a District basis. However, as there were in England and Wales, at the time of writing of the Report (September, 1973), 218 Districts and only 585 whole time equivalent (w.t.e.) clinical psychologists, District organization was ruled out as a general solution for the time being, although 'in the longer term there may be scope for moving towards a District-based service' (para. 5.3.1). Secondly, although the above discussion refers to decisions being made by 'the Department', they would of course be made by individual, or groups of, clinical psychologists. *Which* individuals or groups will depend upon the internal organization of the Department, to be discussed below. Thirdly, 'Area Department' was intended to be an organizational, and not a physical, construction. Although the Report did recommend (para. 5.3.8) that Area Departments should have a defined headquarters in addition to offices and laboratories in those units which it serves, an actual building was neither a necessary nor a sufficient feature — a point which surprisingly often has been misunderstood.

*Specialist sections*

The second Recommendation concerning the unit into which services should be organized was that Area Departments should comprise a number of specialist sections each appropriate to a different field of work (para. 5.3.4.). It was proposed that a fully-developed Area Department might contain eight specialist groupings: (1) physical handicap, (2) mental handicap, (3) child health (child psychiatry and paediatrics), (4) neurological sciences (neurology and neurosurgery), (5) mental illness (including forensic psychiatry and psychotherapy), (6) geriatrics, (7) adolescent services, and (8) primary health care.

Although the Departments as a whole would thus be comprehensive and 'generic', it was not intended that their *individual members* would be generic Jacks and Jills of all trades; rather, the organization would enable, and even encourage, clinical psychologists to specialize in work with specific client groups.

The eight specialist groupings listed were only suggestions and a list drawn up today would certainly include general medicine and surgery, and possibly health education and preventive medicine. However, in this and in other respects, the Report stressed 'the need for flexibility and for local arrangements to take account of local needs'.

**Growth of Area and District Departments**

Although no formal survey has been carried out, it appears that by 1982 most NHS clinical psychologists were members of Departments whose organization of services had been influenced to some extent by the Trethowan recommendations.

There were some Departments, based either on an Area or a District, which had all the organizational features noted above as characterizing the Trethowan-style Departments. A few of these had been in existence for several years, since some localities had anticipated the Trethowan recommendations; for example, Tayside Area Department was established in 1972. However, few of these Departments provided more than three or four of the possible specialist services recommended in the Report. Where Area or District Departments of this sort had been set up, a clinical psychologist had usually been appointed to be Head of Department (usually titled 'Area Psychologist' or 'District Psychologist') whose Job Description normally made him/her responsible to the Authority for the administration of the Department, and for the co-ordination, development, and promotion of standards of its professional work. More common than fully-integrated Trethowan-style Departments were what are best termed Area or District *services* — loose federations of Departments within an Area or District which, while maintaining their independence, internal administrative structure and contractual links with specific hospitals, agreed to co-operate in the Area or District-wide planning and co-ordinating of clinical services and training. A clinical psychologist was often appointed, or in some cases elected by peers, to facilitate this co-operation and to carry out some duties for the Authority; these psychologists were usually described as 'Area (or District) Co-ordinators of Psychological Services'.

**Evaluation of Trethowan Recommendations**

By 1980, there had been sufficient experience of Trethowan-style Departments for the British Psychological Society to be able to attempt their evaluation. Four main advantages were noted.

(i) *Flexibility*. Possibly the major advantage indicated by experience was flexibility in the use of the main resource of the Department, which is psychologists' time. Departments organized in line with the Trethowan Recommendations appear to be better able to allocate their resources according to their assessment of the needs of the population served. Individual clinical psychologists are not tied contractually to some specific hospitals or services when, in their judgement, they might have made a more effective contribution elsewhere. Thus: 'it is becoming common for individuals with specialist skills to have both hospital and community duties, or to work across two or more sites' (BPS, 1980). There are other aspects of flexibility to which the BPS might have referred. Posts which fall vacant can be reallocated from one speciality to another, if the Department considers that this would provide a more effective use of resources. Further, this flexibility enables psychologists to adopt new models of professional practice, such as the 'corporate practice' model with its emphasis on the execution of defined projects by *ad hoc* teams of psychologists, advocated by Hawks (1981) as one solution to the manpower shortage.

(ii) *Exchange of ideas*. The second major advantage noted by the BPS was that these Departments promoted closer contacts, and hence greater exchange of ideas and information, among clinical psychologists specializing in different fields. Methods developed primarily for use with one client group are often found to be applicable to others.

(iii) *Professional support*. Thirdly, where such Departments do not exist, it frequently happens that relatively inexperienced clinical psychologists are appointed to posts in which they are single-handed and professionally isolated. This is particularly common where services are being expanded to a new speciality or locality. The BPS considered that this frequently leads to problems of poor morale, which in turn '. . . have led to heavy wastage from the profession, especially at Basic Grade'. By contrast, in Trethowan-style Departments, individual clinical psychologists have access to the professional and administrative advice and support of a number of colleagues, who often collectively have a wide range of experience. The BPS also believes that the isolation in which clinical psychologists frequently work make professional standards difficult to maintain: 'We have the impression that even now it is psychologists in those places where Area or District services have not been established who tend to run into professional and administrative problems concerning the services they provide or the way in which they provide them.'

(iv) *Professional standards*. Finally, in the opinion of the BPS, these Departments have 'made the organization of clinical psychology training much more efficient and are believed to have contributed to a raising of standards'. This is the case not only with pre-qualification ('Probationer') training but also at the post-qualification level, at which Area or District organization permits Basic or Senior Grade psychologists to obtain, if they wish, experience of several specialities without the need to change job.

(v) *Multidisciplinary teamwork.* A fifth point should be made. Experience has shown that there is no incompatibility between a clinical psychologist belonging to an Area or District Department and becoming closely involved in the day-to-day work of a specific hospital or multidisciplinary team. Because individual (qualified) clinical psychologists are not accountable on matters of 'purely professional judgement' (see below), and are thus able to make decisions about their patients without necessarily obtaining the approval of a senior psychologist colleague, they can play a full part in the work of a clinical team. Moreover, belonging to an Area Department does not absolve the individual psychologist from responsibilities to the team; he/she will for example be expected to conform to its clinical policies. Of course, it may occasionally happen that, over some matter, the policies of the Clinical Psychology Department conflict with the policies of the clinical team to which a member of that Department belongs. If such disagreement cannot be resolved by discussion, it is the responsibility of the individual psychologist to do whatever, in his/her judgement, is in the best interests of the client, preferably after having sought the advice of an experienced, independent colleague.

## Effects of the 1982 Reorganization

The steady progress towards the development of Trethowan-style Departments was interrupted by the 1982 NHS reorganization. At the time of writing (July, 1982), the full implications are not yet apparent, but they may well be serious for several small professions, including clinical psychology.

The major problem is the low number of clinical psychologists. The abolition of the Area tier will mean that services will have to be based on Districts. However, one quarter of the new DHAs will have no qualified clinical psychologists at all; another quarter will have three or fewer (w.t.e.) in post. Few, even of the best-staffed Districts, will be able to provide anything like the range of specialist services envisaged in the Trethowan Report. (The effects of reorganization in Scotland and Wales will be slight, since Areas have been retained.)

Before discussing possible solutions to the problems created by the 1982 reorganization, it will be helpful to identify those features of the comprehensive, integrated Departments proposed in the Trethowan Report which are particularly important to preserve in any new set of arrangements. Three may be considered. The first is that services should be organized on the basis of a population rather than an institution; rather than, that the terms of reference of the Department should be to provide a service to the population of a locality, rather than to a specific hospital. The BPS (1980) states unequivocally that:

'reversion to Departments based on individual hospitals would severely damage the quality of services provided . . .'. A second is that Departments should be generic, with psychologists from different specialities working alongside one another. The third reflects the potentially important role of the Head of Department as a District Officer. The Trethowan Report envisaged that the Head of the Area Department would regularly co-operate with other Area Officers in the detailed planning of a wide range of services, not only those directly affecting clinical psychology. The experience of recent years has provided many examples of how skilled and experienced clinical psychologists have had a significant influence on the provision of services for a variety of client groups, and of the importance of psychological factors being considered when plans for facilities and services are being drawn up. Since the 1982 reorganization, it has been the District level at which it is important for clinical psychologists to be influential. Whatever arrangements are made, it is essential that some psychologist or psychologists should be delegated to undertake these duties, and should be given time off from other tasks to enable him/her/them to do so.

The BPS (1980) proposed two solutions to the problem of providing the comprehensive and integrated range of services envisaged in the Trethowan Report in a two-tier (Regions and Districts) health service. One was to organize services on a Regional basis, so as to bring together in one Trethowan-style Department a mean of sixty qualified clinical psychologists (1980 figures, range 33–102) of different specializations, who would organize their services Region-wide. Although this model is adopted by some highly specialized branches of medicine and surgery, and has attractive features, it did not commend itself to the Secretary of State, since one of the intentions in the reorganization was to strengthen local (i.e., DHA) control over services.

An alternative is to base services on the District, but to make arrangements for the sharing of services across District boundaries so that, for example, a clinical psychologist employed by one DHA might spend some sessions weekly in an adjoining District, with the latter refunding the employing DHA a proportion of his/her salary and expenses. However, for such 'agency' arrangements to be effective requires machinery to permit the comprehensive planning of services across several DHAs, so that developments in any one DHA would take account of the needs of the others. Methods also have to be found for advising those DHAs which have no experienced clinical psychologists in post. In this connection, the BPS (1980) emphasizes the importance of Regional Clinical Psychology Advisory Committees, and recommends that a psychologist should be designated to undertake the necessary liaison work among the DHAs and between DHAs and RHAs. However, even with effective machinery of this sort, 'agency' arrangements seem certain to discourage the flexible use of manpower which is possibly the main advantage of Trethowan-style Departments.

## INTERNAL ORGANIZATION OF CLINICAL PSYCHOLOGY DEPARTMENTS

The Trethowan Report also made recommendations about the internal management structure of Area Departments, that is about the formal roles and relationships which should exist among the individual members of the Department. Although referring to Area Departments, these Recommendations apply equally to the new District Departments. To avoid confusion, the original 'Area' terminology will be used in the following sections.

### Trethowan Recommendations

The major proposals were as follows —

*Head of department.* Para. 5.3.6 recommended that a psychologist should be appointed to be Head of the Area Clinical Psychology Department, who would have 'the major responsibility for its overall co-ordination and development'. Although the post would not primarily be administrative, he/she 'would clearly be the key figure in the general development of clinical psychology services'.

*Head of specialist services.* A second Recommendation was that in these duties, the Head of the Area Department would be assisted by a psychologist in each of the specialist services who 'would have overall responsibility, under the head of department, for the general development in the Area of his specialized element of the clinical psychology service' (para. 5.3.4).

### Discussion

These Recommendations, in particular the former, generated considerable controversy and misunderstanding, and several points need to be discussed here.

#### *Appointment of psychologist*

First, it should not go unremarked that para. 5.3.6 specified that the Head of Department should be a psychologist. Only a few years ago, in many parts of the country, it was taken for granted that clinical psychologists should be administratively and professionally accountable to doctors. This Recommendation derives from an earlier one in the Report, that clinical psychologists in the NHS 'should be regarded as having full professional status' (para. 5.2.2). One aspect of this status is that it is inappropriate for the professional work of a clinical psychologist to be managed and directed by a non-psychologist.

*Duties of head of department*

Although the Report did not specify the duties of the Head of the Area Department, it appears that three types were envisaged.

(i) *Administrative duties.* These would include ensuring that Department members were aware of, and conformed to, their conditions of employment, and NHS regulations such as those to do with health and safety; controlling the budgets for the purchase of equipment and supplies, and possibly also for salaries and travelling expenses; ensuring the safe keeping and maintenance of equipment; and so on. These administrative duties would, in normal NHS manner, be delegated to the Head of Department by the Area Administrator, who would be ultimately responsible and to whom, for these duties, the Head of Department would be accountable.

(ii) *Professional duties.* The Head of Department would also have responsibilities for the professional work of the Department. He/she would be required to *co-ordinate its professional services*, for example by ensuring that duties and resources were shared out among the various clinical psychologists so as to provide the most effective and efficient service possible, in line with overall Area policy. Other professional duties would involve the monitoring of the needs of the population, and the presentation to the Authority of detailed proposals for the *development of clinical psychology* and related services to meet these needs. Other duties would concern *professional standards and development.* The Authority would expect the Head of Department to ensure that the work of the Department was being carried out to acceptable professional standards, that good practice was being promoted, and that individual clinical psychologists had access to appropriate training and counselling about their professional work and careers. The Report anticipated that, in respect of these professional duties, the Head of Department would work closely with the Area Medical Officer.

(iii) *Duties as an Area Officer.* In addition to these administrative and professional duties, the Head of Department would also be expected to undertake some important activities in his/her capacity as an Area Officer. Thus, he/she might co-operate with other Area Officers in the detailed co-ordination and forward planning of a wide range of Area services, whose scope might extend well beyond clinical psychology, for example the development of comprehensive services for the elderly, or the planning of a programme of health education.

*Accountability for personal professional work*

Perhaps the most controversial and confusing part of the Trethowan Report was about whether individual clinical psychologists should be accountable to the Head of Department on matters of 'purely professional judgement'. The Report makes contradictory recommendations. In the text (para. 5.3.6) it states that '. . . below Principal level . . . all clinical psychologists should be directly accountable to a professional superior' whereas in the Summary this is changed to '. . . members of the Department should *not* have to account to (the Head) on matters of purely professional judgement' (emphasis added).

'Professional judgement' refers to decisions made by an individual clinical psychologist about his/her professional work — assessing and treating patients, training staff, etc. Being 'accountable' means that A (the person to whom B is professionally accountable) is entitled to assign work to B, to issue specific instructions about the goals to be achieved and the methods to be used, and to assess the quality and effectiveness of B's work. This is the sort of accountability which a trainee psychologist has to a supervisor, and which qualified members of some professions such as nursing have to senior colleagues. A recommendation that Basic and Senior Grade clinical psychologists should be accountable professionally to a 'superior' would thus have major implications for the organization of clinical psychology services. However, it appears that the final intention of the Trethowan Committee was reflected in the Summary rather than the text.

Although the Trethowan Report thus did not recommend that Heads of Area Departments should 'manage' the professional work of their junior staff, the Report clearly indicates that they should 'monitor' their work. Thus, a Head of Department is expected to obtain sufficient information to be able to satisfy him/herself that the personal professional work of each member of the Department is in accordance with accepted professional practice and standards, and conforms to Department and Authority policy.

## Discussion

The role of Head of Department was of course well-established long before the publication of the Trethowan Report: almost all NHS clinical psychology Departments, whether Area or District or site-based, have a senior member designated Head of Department. However, the publication of the Report stimulated a debate within the profession about the duties, and more especially the appropriate limits of the authority, of the Head of Department, and about the viability of alternative modes of organization.

### *Evaluation of Trethowan recommendations*

The Trethowan proposal that the administrative and professional organization of the Department should be made the responsibility of one appointed clinical psychologist, who would be the most senior member of the Department, has some advantages. It is probably the most efficient method. It also appeals to employing Authorities, who can ensure that the running of the Department is in the hands of someone of their own choosing, who is (presumably) of appropriate experience and ability.

The fear is sometimes expressed that these arrangements would concentrate too much power in the hands of one individual. However, some of the responsibilities of a Head of Department are those which he/she exercises directly on behalf of the Authority. They are thus clearly defined, highly circumscribed and not subject to personal whim: examples of this type of responsibility are ensuring that Department members do not claim excessive travel expenses and that they perform the sorts of duties specified in their Job Descriptions. The other main responsibilities of a Head of Department are 'professional' and can be summarized as 'promoting the work of the Department'. In connection with these, neither the NHS nor the profession expects the Head to 'manage' the work of colleagues, or to insist that specific activities are carried out. Here, the appropriate relationship between the Head and the members of the Department is a 'co-ordinating' one, with the Head ensuring, for example, that procedures for organizing work and for monitoring standards are agreed, and that obstacles to the implementation of these procedures are overcome. Of course, the disciplinary procedures of the NHS can be used by a Head of Department against a psychologist who appears, through incapacity or malice, to be obstructing the work of the Department. Again, there are clear safeguards against the abuse of such procedures, one of which is the entitlement of Department members to invoke the NHS grievance procedure against a Head who appears to be acting unreasonably.

There are potential disadvantages also. An ineffective or insensitive Head can have a damaging effect on the work of his/her colleagues. Secondly, the Head has to reconcile two sets of responsibilities, to the Authority and to his psychologist colleagues, which may be incompatible. For example, the Authority may instruct the Head of Department to reduce the costs of the clinical psychology service, at a time when the psychologists in the Department wish to encourage expansion. Thirdly, the designation of the most senior psychologist in a Department as 'Head of Department', and the grading structure with its four levels (see below), often mislead colleagues in other professions into believing that clinical psychology is more hierarchical than in fact it is. Thus, District Officers or consultants often expect a Head of Department to be answerable for clinical decisions made by members of the Department and to have authority to 'manage' these decisions, in the same way as consultants 'manage' the clinical work of their registrars. Again, the Head may find him/herself having to reconcile the incompatible views of the members of the Department and of senior colleagues in other professions.

### *Other possible arrangements*

Other arrangements for the management of administrative and professional duties within a Department are of course possible. However, it should be realized that within a highly structured organization such as the NHS, only quite small variations in arrangements are possible. Thus, employing Authorities will always make arrangements for each of their employees to be administratively, and where appropriate professionally, accountable to an Officer of the Authority. *Someone* is responsible for ensuring that each employee is aware of, and conforms to, the administrative arrangements of the Authority (conditions of service, health and safety regulations, etc.) and for ensuring that his/her professional duties are performed efficiently, in accordance with Authority policy and accepted professional standards. Similarly, arrangements are always made for ensuring that the work of a group of employees, for example members of a Department, is co-ordinated, that resources are allocated appropriately, etc. The specific arrangements which are made by the Authority will vary according to local circumstances, and the professional and occupational group involved, but some arrangements are always made. Because the accountability of the clinical psychologist has not in the past always been made explicit, some members of the profession have been misled into believing that no such arrangements exist, and that the Trethowan Report somehow forced an autocratic structure on a profession which was previously untrammelled by bureaucracy. On the contrary, arrangements for accountability have always existed and NHS clinical psychologists have no choice about *whether* to be accountable, although they may be able to influence the *specific* arrangements which are made.

Some well-publicized Departments have claimed to have democratized themselves by abolishing the post of Head of Department. In practice, what appears to have happened is that those administrative and professional duties which were previously carried out by the Head (a psychologist) have merely been transferred to an administrator (a non-psychologist). There may be advantages in such a transfer, but it is not immediately obvious that they include greater democracy. Other Departments have replaced an appointed Head with one elected by the Department. Although this has some merit, there are few Departments with sufficient psychologists with the necessary experience and interest to make an election more than a formality.

Medicine provides an instructive model. In the NHS, administration and the details of planning are the responsibility of appointed Officers (DMOs etc.) whereas the organization and development of clinical services within the overall strategy of the District is the function of the clinicians themselves, operating through 'cogwheel' Divisions and their elected chairmen. This model also has many merits, but again the problem is mainly one of small numbers. Few Districts have enough psychologists to justify such an arrangement.

Possibly the most satisfactory system, given the existing size and relative lack of experience of the profession, is to have an appointed Head of Department, but to ensure that adequate arrangements exist both for the Head, and for the Authority and its Officers, to take account of the advice of other members of the Department.

## FOUR RELATED ISSUES

This section will consider four issues related to the organization of clinical psychology services; they are dealt with together for no reason other than convenience.

## Grading Structure

The grading structure of clinical psychologists, as for most NHS employees, is determined by the Whitley Council system of collective bargaining, by which pay and conditions of employment are negotiated nationally by management and staff side representatives. The structure for clinical psychologists has four grades — Basic (divided into probationary and post-probationary periods), Senior, Principal, and Top (divided into those with, and without, greater responsibilities). It is important to realize that a grade, *by itself*, does not necessarily have managerial implications, and that the designation of someone as, for example, Top or Principal grade does not give that person authority over someone designated Senior or Basic grade. Any administrative or professional responsibility which one psychologist has to or for another can be given only by the employing Authority (DHA) and must be specified in the Job Descriptions of those concerned.

However, since the publication of the Trethowan Report, attempts have been made to relate grading to administrative responsibilities. These attempts culminated in the revised grading definitions of Principal and Top Grade posts, published in March, 1982. Thus, of the four alternative criteria of Principal Psychologist, only one refers to expertise in clinical work or research. The other three are administrative — head of a hospital department, head of a specialist section within a department of psychology, or head of a District service. Similarly, while Top Grade posts may be awarded to psychologists on the basis of their distinguished clinical or research contribution to clinical psychology, it is clear that such appointments will be exceptional, and that the majority of Top Grade posts will be justified because of their managerial responsibilities.

These new grading definitions will of course make even more difficult any attempts to devise alternative methods, of the sort discussed in the previous section, of organizing clinical psychology departments.

## Advisory Committees

A clear distinction must be made between the management and the advisory structures of the NHS. Regional and District Officers, including District Psychologists, are part of the management structure, and an important part of their job is to act on behalf of their Authorities to ensure that other NHS employees are aware of, and conform to, the administrative and professional policies and regulations of the Authorities. However, the 1974 reorganization also made important provision for professional staff to *advise* the Authorities about what these professional policies should be. This is done by means both of a network of advisory committees representing specific professions and of multidisciplinary health care planning teams advising on services for particular client groups. Advice of this sort can be very important because of the flexibility permitted to each RHA and DHA in the interpretation of policies determined at 'higher' levels, and in the allocation of resources. Of course, the appointed officers can also advise the Authorities, and through their close contacts with the Authorities, and their access to information, may often exert more influence than the advisory committees.

With regard to clinical psychology, although the Trethowan Report recommended that the Head of the Area Department was to be 'regarded as the spokesman for clinical psychologists in the Area', the Report also recommended that 'the views of clinical psychologists as a profession should be taken fully into account in the planning and operation of Area services', and that Area Clinical Psychology Advisory Committees should be established in those Areas where the service was sufficiently developed to justify them. It further recommended that Regional Advisory Committees should also be established, and that advice should be available nationally, to the DHSS.

A recent unpublished survey showed that in almost every Region, and in many Districts, in England, Clinical Psychology Advisory Committees had been set up. However, although the 1973 NHS Reorganization Act enabled the Secretary of State to recognize the advisory committees of health professions (and required him to recognize those of doctors and nurses), no clinical psychology advisory committee has been so recognized.

The effectiveness of these Clinical Psychology Advisory Committees varies greatly. While some — a few — are regularly consulted by their Authorities on matters such as service development and resource allocation, many have little contact with them, and seem to provide little more than a forum for clinical psychologists to exchange information and to co-ordinate training and occasionally services. These are useful enough activities, but are not the main purpose of Advisory Committees, which is to influence the decisions of Health Authorities. The important potential role of Regional Advisory Committees in influencing those DHAs which employ few, or no, experienced clinical psychologists has already been noted. The situation in Scotland and Wales is better, and both have national consultative committees which, being statutory, routinely advise on a wide range of topics. In England such advice is given by the Consultant Adviser to the Chief Medical Officer at the DHSS.

## Manpower Planning

Although staffing is the responsibility of the Authorities, the DHSS can exert influence through the operation of nationally-agreed norms. Expressed as a ratio of the general population, these norms indicate for various professions either the minimum acceptable level of staffing or the desirable level of staffing. These norms also influence training and, for example, the intake to medical schools is adjusted to take account of medical manpower norms. However, no agreed norms exist for clinical psychology, so that Authorities are under no pressure from DHSS to employ a given number of psychologists.

Thus, large variations exist between Regions — ranging from one qualified psychologist per 37,000 population to one per 77,000 — and between Districts, with some better than one per 20,000 and many with no clinical psychologists at all. Furthermore, there is no formal link between manpower needs and the provision and funding of training places. It would seem to be important that both at national, and at Regional, level a coherent manpower strategy should be agreed which would balance supply of, and demand for, clinical psychologists and would reduce the discrepancies in staffing levels between Regions and specialities.

**NHS and Local Authorities**

Major problems arise in the provision of services because of the division of responsibilities between the NHS and local authorities, which are financed and managed quite independently of one another. It is the latter, through their Social Services departments, which are responsible for personal social services and for the community and residential care of such groups as children, the elderly, the physically and mentally handicapped, and patients discharged from psychiatric hospitals. Few local authorities employ clinical psychologists, and an organizational problem for NHS Clinical Psychology Departments is how to ensure that services can be provided for those clients who, although technically not the responsibility of the NHS, would benefit from clinical psychology advice and intervention — and might indeed have so benefited before their discharge from hospital. Various solutions are being tried out, such as the joint funding by Health Authorities and local authorities of clinical psychology posts, and the secondment of NHS clinical psychologists. While the 1974 reorganization encouraged such arrangements, for example by making local authority and AHA boundaries co-terminous, serious problems are likely to be caused by the 1982 reorganization of the NHS since each local authority will now have to relate to several DHAs.

In addition, many clinical psychologists come into contact with educational psychologists employed by local authorities. The Court Report (1976) referred to ways in which clinical and educational psychologists could co-operate in the provision of child health services, and the BPS Working Party on Psychological Services for Children (1981) proposed that Area Groups of Psychological Services for Children should be set up in each locality, to facilitate the integration of the services provided by clinical and educational psychologists.

The 1982 reorganization will impede co-operation between clinical and educational psychology departments, just as it will between clinical psychology and social service departments. It is important that in the next few years methods should be found to facilitate the provision of NHS clinical psychology services across NHS-local authority boundaries, and to ensure co-ordination with other services.

## IMPLICATIONS FOR THE INDIVIDUAL

The way in which services will in future be organized is thus by no means certain. In addition to the continuing debate over the internal organization of Departments, the 1982 NHS reorganization threatens to retard by many years the development of those integrated, population-based Departments offering a comprehensive range of services which experience has suggested offer many advantages to clients and psychologists alike. A further threat is posed by the Nodder Report (1980) on the organization and management of mental illness hospitals. If fully implemented, the proposals of the Report might lead to the strengthening of the management of mental hospitals but at the expense of integration of the psychiatric sector with other parts of the District. While there would be many advantages to such proposals, they are likely to make the maintenance of generic District Departments of clinical psychology still more difficult.

In the face of this uncertainty some clinical psychologists will be tempted to ignore problems of organization and occupy themselves wholly with their own clients or research. This would be irresponsible, for two reasons. First, it is simply not possible to be an effective clinician in the NHS without having a detailed knowledge of management and organizational relationships. No NHS clinical psychologist works wholly in isolation, and even those who are not members of multidisciplinary teams must regularly interact with other psychologists and members of related professions. All too frequently, the clinical effectiveness of a psychologist is reduced by the apparently thoughtless actions of colleagues, which however in turn are often the result of the failure of the clinical psychologist to understand the roles and responsibilities of other professions, to consult the appropriate committee or (in the immortal words of the MMPI) to find out 'who should be gotten next to'.

However secondly, and more generally, if the scientific evidence has led clinical psychologists to conclude that our methods are capable of playing a significant part in preventing and reducing psychological disorder and distress — and this book provides such evidence — then individual practitioners have a professional obligation to ensure that these methods are made available, efficiently and effectively, to as many as possible of those clients who would benefit from them. This will be achieved only if appropriate forms of service delivery are developed and implemented. Indeed, it may not be just a matter of improving services, but one of retaining existing levels of provision. In the conditions of financial stringency which are likely to exist in the NHS in the foreseeable future, there will be great competition for resources by the various professions and services. It will be those which are poorly organized, use their existing resources inefficiently and ineffectively, and whose voice is not heard when decisions are made, which will be most at risk. Unless clinical psychology solves its organizational problems, it may well find itself starved of resources, until the work of individual practitioners is jeopardized, and the future of the profession as a whole is threatened. Clinical psychologists should devote as much thought, effort and initiative to developing appropriate forms of organization as they do to devising new methods of treatment and assessment, for without the former, the latter may remain unused.

## ACKNOWLEDGEMENTS

I am grateful to Annette Meadows for helpful comments on a draft of this chapter.

## REFERENCES

British Psychological Society (1980). *Comments on the DHSS Consultative Paper 'Patients First'*. Leicester: BPS.

British Psychological Society (1981). *Report of a Working Party on Psychological Services for Children.* Leicester: BPS.

Court, S. D. (1976). *Fit for the Future*. London: HMSO.

Hawks, D. V. (1981). The dilemma of clinical practice. In I. McPherson and A. Sutton (eds), *Reconstructing Clinical Practice.* London: Croom Helm.

Nodder, T. E. (1980). *Organization and Management Problems of Mental Illness Hospitals: Report of a Working Party.* London: HMSO.

Trethowan, W. H. (1977). *The Role of Psychologists in the Health Services.* London: HMSO.

Zuckerman, S. (1968). *Hospital Scientific and Technical Services.* London: HMSO.

# *PART II*

# Practice of Clinical Psychology in Traditional Settings

The Practice of Clinical Psychology in Great Britain
Edited by A. Liddell


*Chapter 5*

# *Mental illness*

*Fraser N. Watts*

## APPROACHES TO ASSESSMENT AND FORMULATION

For many clinical psychologists the concept of mental illness is itself a controversial one. To have an illness often suggests having a group of symptoms that regularly occur together, have a common cause (normally a biological one) and have a predictable course and response to treatment. How far is this true of the conditions presented by psychiatric patients? There are at least two factors that tend to cloud debate on this question. One is a tendency to accept the concept of mental illness for either *all* psychiatric patients or for *none*. If the question is being approached on scientific grounds, each putative 'mental illness' has to be examined individually. Few would deny, for example, that a better case can be made out for manic-depressive psychosis as a mental illness than for personality disorder. One indication of this is the far better agreement that can be obtained between different clinicians in diagnosing the former. Such differences between the status of psychiatric conditions can be formalized by arranging them in a hierarchical model (Foulds and Bedford, 1975). Another factor that clouds the debate is the adoption of a rigid and idealized concept of what is an 'illness', that would be untenable in general medicine let alone in psychiatry. Buss (1966) among others has drawn attention to the diverse ways in which the concept of illness can be used, to the differences for example between infectious and systemic diseases. When these two considerations are fully appreciated, it becomes difficult to justify on scientific and logical grounds the firm and sweeping stances that are sometimes taken up, either for or against the concept of mental illness.

There is a separate set of issues about the practical implications of the concept of mental illness. The well-known attack that Szasz (1961) has mounted is largely made on such grounds. To call someone mentally ill can suggest to the person concerned that he has neither control over his condition nor responsibility for it. It can also justify in others attitudes and behaviour, whether coercive or paternalistic, that exacerbate the condition. These dangers are real enough, but they are not necessary consequences of careful use of the concept of mental illness. In addition, there are pragmatic questions for the clinician about whether the concept of mental illness helps or hinders in formulating a clinicial problem and making an appropriate intervention. The balance of advantage here may depend on the kind of interventions a particular clinician has at his disposal. For pharmacological methods of treatment, it may be useful to think in terms of categories of mental illness. However, for psychological interventions, it has less value. Clinical psychologists are probably justified in concluding that whatever the arguments for or against the concept of mental illness in other contexts, for them it is of little professional value. However, there are exceptions even to this conclusion. In particular it is important to be aware that the best approach to a common presenting problem may depend on the context of other symptoms in which it occurs. For example, avoidance of social situations may need to be approached differently when it occurs in the context of paranoid delusions from when it occurs in the context of generalized anxiety.

Because clinical psychologists have found concepts of mental illness of little professional value, they have become increasingly reluctant to spend time using psychometric methods to try to decide whether or not a patient has a particular category of mental illness. It is also relevant that efforts to develop valid diagnostic tools have been strikingly unsuccessful. There have been repeated attempts to develop psychometric tests of thought disorder that will be an aid in the diagnosis of schizophrenia (Chapman and Chapman, 1973). These tests have had various focuses over the decades. Some have tried to assess 'concrete' thinking, some 'over-inclusive' thinking, while most recently Bannister has developed a test of thought disorder within the framework of Kelly's personal construct theory. The reasons why attempts to develop valid diagnostic tests have generally been unsuccessful are no doubt complex, but one crucial consideration is that tests which have initially seemed promising when applied to clear criterion groups have subsequently been applied to borderline cases, where their validity has been less satisfactory.

An alternative assessment approach has sought, rather than to assign patients to diagnostic categories, to place them on general dimensions of individual differences that basic psychological research has identified in the normal population. An example is the Eysenck Personality Questionnaire that assesses the dimensions of extraversion, neuroticism, and psychoticism that have been identified by factor analysis (Eysenck, 1970). Other personality questionnaires measure personality dimensions that have been arrived at on more general theoretical considerations rather than empirical research, such as the Edwards Personal Preference Schedule. A limitation with all questionnaires that measure general traits is that they may not describe the personality of an individual patient with sufficient validity to be useful for clinical purposes. A higher degree of validity is required in assessing an individual than in comparing contrasting groups of people in research. There is the additional problem that personality functioning is variable across situations (Mischel, 1968), and measures of general traits do not offer this kind of differentiation. Assessments of intelligence, another general dimension of individual differences, also have limited clinical usefulness for similar reasons. They seldom allow clinically relevant criterion variables to be predicted with sufficient precision to be of practical value. Comparisons of performance on various different intellectual tasks may be useful in neuropsychological assessment, but that is a different use of the test materials (see Chapter 8).

Rather than assigning psychiatric patients to diagnostic categories, or placing them on general personality dimensions, most clinical psychologists have preferred to focus their attention on a single presenting problem and assess this thoroughly. The methods of assessment that are now used predominantly reflect this approach. What are needed are techniques that will enable the psychologist to *assess the severity* of a presenting problem and to *analyse its determinants*. Direct observations of behaviour and structured interviewing have generally proved better adapted to this purpose than standard psychometric instruments.

Typically, in the initial assessment of a problem, these methods are used to investigate conditions that contribute to its genesis or maintenance. An example will make clear what this involves. Slade (1972) has reported an investigation of a patient presenting with hallucinations. The hallucinations were not present continuously, and the aim of the investigation was to identify factors that differentiated times when they were present and absent. Three times a day the patient completed a record of the hallucinations during the preceding part of the day. He also rated various dimensions of his emotional state, and environmental variables such as the number of people present and the noise level. The most striking finding was that hallucinations were associated with high levels of anxiety and tension. Subsequent enquiries revealed that these anxieties were largely related to the patient's home life and family. Treatment of this produced a marked reduction in hallucinations. The ratings also revealed a less pronounced tendency for the hallucinations to be associated with lack of engagement in activity, a finding which was followed up in subsequent research.

This illustrates the analysis of how clinically relevant variables covary over time. Alternatively the analysis may focus on sequences, usually on identifying what regularly precedes or succeeds the problem behaviour. This was an element in a case study of a depressed patient reported by Lewinsohn and Shaw (1969). The patient was depressed and had various other problems such as fainting spells, a stiff neck, and a preoccupation with a brain tumour. However, the psychologists decided to focus on inequalities in marital interaction. Their home observations showed that in conversation, the time spent on the husband's interests was three times that spent on the wife's. Further analysis showed that when the husband opened up a topic, the wife was more likely to listen attentively and continue the topic than vice-versa (i.e. the husband attending to the wife). By changing these patterns of reacting to each other's conversation, so as to increase the number of positive reactions shown in *both* directions, the imbalance in the distribution of conversation time was rectified. The successful course of therapy seemed to vindicate the initial decision to focus on marital interaction rather than the wife's somatic complaints.

If such investigations are to arrive at the important determinants of presenting problems efficiently, the clinical psychologist needs to make good use of his clinical experience, his scientific knowledge of psychopathology and his understanding of general psychological processes. Any of these may be a source of fruitful hypotheses. It is not always necessary for the data on which such an analysis is based to be collected through direct observation. Hypotheses about variables associated with problem behaviours can also form the basis of a structured interview in which the patient himself provides the relevant data. This is obviously a less time-consuming method of investigation, though it introduces risks of distortion and concealment.

Methods are also available for the assessment of cognitive variables surrounding a presenting clinical problem (e.g. Merluzzi *et al.*, 1981). One of these which is well established is the use of Kelly's Repertory Grid Test to assess how a patient construes relevant aspects of the environment (Bannister and Fransella, 1971). For example, it may be relevant to understanding the behaviour of an anorexic patient who diets to a pathologically excessive degree, to know how she perceives fat and thin people generally, what is associated in her conceptual structure with fatness and thinness, and who have been the significant fat and thin people in her life from whom these assumptions are probably derived. An investigation of these cognitive structures can also provide a valuable explanation of the presenting problem that leads to an intervention aimed at reviewing and changing maladaptive cognitive structures.

Finally, methods are available for monitoring changes in the severity of particular problems. Many checklists and rating scales are available for particular problems (Barlow, 1981). Techniques are available too for monitoring changes in the unique complaints of individual patients such as Shapiro's personal questionnaire method (Shapiro, 1961).

In general it is the style of clinical psychologists' approach to assessment to make good use of systematic methods of collecting information, and to obtain relevant objective information wherever possible. This parallels, in the clinical situation, the objective approach to psychological phenomena that characterizes basic psychological science. However, clinical psychologists inevitably also have to make use of more intuitive judgements about clinical problems and relatively subjective inferences from the available information. Not to do so would be to fail to make use of the highly efficient information processing of which the human mind is capable. The problem lies in the bias and error which subjective judgements may introduce. A balance needs to be kept between objective methods and intuitive judgements (Watts, 1980).

## BEHAVIOURAL APPROACHES TO CLINICAL INTERVENTIONS

The approach to intervention most commonly used by psychologists is the behavioural one. The most important features of this are those relating to its general methodological style. The therapeutic intervention characteristically focuses on specific problems that are identified before treatment begins. In many other kinds of psychological therapy the joint exploration of the presenting problem by the patient and therapist is a key part of the therapy itself. The behavioural approach makes it easier to select an intervention which is specifically geared to the presenting problem. For this reason there is no single method of behaviour therapy but a series of methods designed for specific problems (Turner *et al*., 1981). Another scientific advantage of the behavioural approach is that because the target problem can be specified more clearly before treatment begins, it is easier to obtain a measure of the severity of the problem at this stage and then to monitor changes as a result of treatment.

Behavioural treatments for anxiety and related problems are among the most commonly used. Anxiety can be experienced directly in the forms of anxious thoughts or of somatic symptoms. Common indirect effects of anxiety are phobic avoidance behaviour and compulsive rituals. For each of these problems, interventions of recognized effectiveness have been developed.

The best developed approach to anxious thoughts is the self-instruction method developed by Meichenbaum (1977). Anxiety is often manifested in negative self-talk, in which people ruminate about the difficult or frightening aspects of a situation. Such anxious self-talk tends to be stereotyped and easily recognized. Meichenbaum's method involves teaching the anxious person to recognize this negative self-talk, to terminate it whenever it begins, and to replace it with some 'coping' self-talk that directs attention to what needs to be done practically to cope with the situation, and also includes an element of encouragement and self-congratulation on success. The technique has been shown to be an effective intervention for specific anxieties, and has the additional merit that once learned it can be employed in any situation that causes anxiety.

If a particular person is more affected by the somatic symptoms of anxiety, the psychologist's intervention can focus on these. The assessment might rely on the patient's self-report of somatic complaints or might involve direct measures of psychophysiological responsiveness (Epstein, 1976). People vary in the response system in which the effects of anxiety is most apparent, such as accelerated heart-beat, increased muscular tension, etc. The intervention could focus on a particular response system, in which case biofeedback might be provided to help train self-regulation of that system. Alternatively training in relaxation could be given that would have a generalized effect on autonomic arousal. Training in the regulation of both self-talk and physiological responsiveness would often be combined in a general programme of anxiety management.

The treatment of phobic avoidance behaviour has a particular historical importance in clinical psychology as Wolpe's (1969) desensitization treatment for this problem was probably the first treatment method to gain widespread usage by British clinical psychologists. The method involves gradual and repeated exposure to an ascending hierarchy of phobic situations under conditions of relaxation that keep the level of anxiety at a minimum. It can be carried out either in the actual situations or in imagination. The record of effectiveness of desensitization with simple phobics is very good, though results are more modest with complex phobias in which there are more likely to be other psychological problems in the background. In general, desensitization has become an exceptionally highly researched, well validated and widely used specific intervention for a mental health problem.

Parallel techniques have been developed for compulsive rituals (Beech and Vaughan, 1978). The key element of treatment involves the controlled prevention, by agreement with the patient, of compulsive rituals such as excessive and meticulous handwashing that are the focus of treatment. Such rituals are typically a response to anxiety about contamination. So, in order to ensure exposure to this anxiety and to provide an opportunity for it to habituate, the patient is first contaminated in whatever way he is anxious about. Often the therapist would act as a 'model' for this and contaminate himself also. Controlled exposure to anxiety arousing cues is the common element in both this procedure and the desensitization of phobic avoidance behaviour.

Similar techniques have been extended to a variety of other emotional problems. An approach to the control of anger has been developed that parallels anxiety management training (Novaco, 1975). Similar techniques have also been developed for the management of depression. The methods of modifying depressive thought developed by Beck *et al.* (1979) are similar to Meichenbaum's method of modifying anxious self-talk. There are also direct methods of modifying the behavioural consequences of depression by, for example, reinstigating potentially rewarding activities. Where the depression arises from an abnormal grief reaction to a bereavement, the grief response can be modified in a way similar to the desensitization of phobic anxiety responses, though it involves more prolonged and intense exposure to the grief (Ramsay, 1979). However, depression seems to lend itself less readily than anxiety to methods of intervention that focus on discrete problems, and the effectiveness of these methods, though promising, requires further investigation (Rehm, 1981).

Much less progress has been made in developing psychological interventions to remedy specific symptoms. Of the work done in this field so far, much has consisted of programmes designed to improve the social functioning of hospital in-patients (discussed later in this chapter). However, some specific methods for psychotic problems are available (Liberman, 1976). The work of Slade on hallucinations already mentioned is one of a number of specific approaches to this disorder. Paranoid delusions are another problem for which a specific method of cognitive therapy has been developed (Milton *et al.*, 1978).

Many psychiatric patients who are not easily classified as having either psychotic or neurotic problems present with a particular behavioural problem, either deviant behaviour that needs to be reduced, or inadequacy of behaviour that needs to be remedied. It is very doubtful whether it is defensible on any grounds to regard such problems as 'mental illness' but they have conventionally been provided for within the framework of the psychiatric services and are conveniently considered here.

Examples of deviant behaviour commonly referred to psychologists are problem drinkers or drug users, sexual deviants, and excessive eaters. In each case specific psychological techniques have been developed which are of some value (Turner *et al.*, 1981) but in each case they have significant limitations. Behavioural methods for problem drinkers and drug users are available that are aimed in some cases at abstinence and in others at controlled usage. Such methods are a valuable adjunct to a general network of services, but are usually not sufficient by themselves. Methods of reducing deviant sexual interests or behaviour probably work best when the client has or can acquire an alternative sex-life that can provide genuine satisfaction and when his motivation for treatment is genuine and not merely a response to social pressure. Psychological treatments for obesity can be effective in those cases where the obesity is due to over-eating. However, psychologists have sometimes been naïve in their assumptions about how often this is the case.

A general approach to improving inadequate social behaviour has been developed, known as social skills training (Trower *et al.*, 1978). The main elements of the programme, as with training in many contexts, are instructions, modelling, rehearsal, and feedback. A crucial preliminary to any such training programme is to identify the aspects of social behaviour to be modified. This is not as straightforward as it may seem as a number of research studies have had difficulty in demonstrating clear differences between socially effective and ineffective groups in the kind of detailed behaviour that can be tackled in a social skills programme. It is often wise to concentrate training efforts on remedying one or two critical areas of inadequate behaviour, rather than to attempt comprehensive retraining. Another potential limitation in social skills training is that the newly acquired behaviour may not generalize to everyday situations, though the psychologist can try to overcome this with carefully devised assignments between training sessions.

Clearly not all these techniques are 'behaviourist' in the sense of focusing exclusively on overt behaviour, but they are 'behavioural' in their methodological style. Behavioural techniques tend to be based on general psychological principles, and in the early days of behaviour therapy learning theory was especially important in generating behavioural methods of therapy. However, it would not be widely recognized that the psychological processes underlying behavioural techniques are more complex than was initially imagined.

## OTHER APPROACHES TO INDIVIDUAL THERAPY

Though the behavioural approach is the one most widely employed by British clinical psychologists, many have had some training in, and experience of, other methods. It is desirable that this should be so. There is growing evidence (e.g., Di Loreto, 1971) that even within a single type of presenting problem the relative effectiveness of different therapeutic approaches depends on the personality of the patient. This means that it is desirable that the psychologist should be competent in a sufficient variety of approaches to be able to use one that is appropriate to each particular patient. An increasing number of psychologists have the skills to do this, though there is a need for more scientifically based guidelines regarding the selection of an appropriate treatment approach.

Many clinicians take the view that the effectiveness of the behavioural methods described so far depend on a good level of motivation and co-operation from the patient. Unfortunately, many patients come to treatment with somewhat mixed motivation. It is in these cases that it seems most important to use other therapeutic methods either to supplement the behavioural approach or as an alternative to it.

One approach which many psychologists would use when there was a need for a broad exploration of a patient's attitude and approach to treatment is 'non-directive' interviewing or counselling. Carl Rogers (1951) has developed a style of interviewing in which the psychologist avoids asking questions, putting forward theoretical formulations of the problem, or in any other way imposing his own frame of reference on the session. Rather the psychologist helps the patient in the task of self-exploration by simply reflecting back to him some key aspects of what he is saying, especially the feeling content. The psychologist strives for a high level of accuracy in these emphatic reflections, and also to show warmth and genuineness to the patient. Rogers suggested that these qualities are fundamental to the effectiveness of any therapy. There is some evidence to support this, though it is not entirely consistent (Mitchell *et al*., 1977). It is not necessary, of course, that this non-directive approach be the sole one used with a patient. An alternative is to use a number of non-directive sessions as a preliminary intervention when the nature of the patient's problem and motivation for change has not become clear through more structured interviewing.

Alternatively, the psychologist can use an explicit theoretical model to explore the patient's motivation and the significance of the problem he presents. The psychodynamic tradition, stemming from Freud but much elaborated by others, is the best established model of this kind, and Malan (1979) has provided a lucid introduction to this. An example of Malan's (pp. 37–39) will give some of the flavour of this approach to the formulation of problems. The patient was depressed and had anxieties about going out. This seemed to be linked to episodes in which everything went red before her eyes. The interviewer decided to explore the possible relevance of the death of the patient's mother, which had occurred two years before. It subsequently emerged that the first attack of seeing red occurred exactly at the second anniversary of the mother's death, though initially the patient was somewhat evasive about the onset of these episodes. The mother had been very dominating and the patient had rebelled against this. Shortly before the mother's death the patient had refused a plea to come and visit her, adding that the mother's worry about her daughter may have been responsible for the stroke of which she died. A link between the attacks of seeing red and the mother's death was established when, well on in the interview, the patient agreed to a suggestion that the attacks were what she imagined the experience of having a stroke to be. Interestingly, this was the point at which she revealed when the attacks had begun. Further links were established when towards the end of the interview it emerged that when the first attack occurred she had felt terrified that she might be driven to commit suicide, and in effect to join her mother in the grave. This made sense of a vague feeling she had mentioned earlier of teetering on the brink of something and just being prevented from falling in. Conflicts about the mother's death were also apparent in repeated guilty dreams in which the mother was still alive and the patient was telling her that she should not be there because she was dead. Treatment consisted of exploration of links between such aspects of the patient's symptoms and history. After five sessions the patient felt much relieved and was able to go back to work.

The psychodynamic approach, like the non-directive one, does not need to be used exclusively with any particular patient. It is possible for a psychologist to use interventions of a structured or behavioural type, but to do so on the basis of an understanding of the patient's psychodynamics. This will particularly guide the way in which specific therapeutic tasks are presented, and help the psychologist to respond appropriately to occasions when the patient does not carry them out. It can also be helpful in understanding the significance of the therapist to the patient. The therapist, whatever method he uses, is likely to become a potent figure in the patient's life and sometimes the object of intense emotions. The nature of these emotions may be influenced by reactions to previous potent figures in the patient's life, especially his parents. This is the essence of the psychodynamic concept of 'transference' (Sandler *et al.*, 1973). To have a framework for understanding the patient's relationship to the therapist can be valuable, whether or not 'interpretations' of this relationship to the patient are used as a central therapeutic technique.

The behavioural, non-directive, and psychodynamic approaches to therapy are three of the more widely used ones, but there are many others (Bannister, 1975) which cannot all be described here. Though each of these has its own ideology and techniques, it is a mistake to emphasize the distinctness of these approaches too much. Therapists with differing orientations show more similarity and overlap in what they actually do with patients than might be supposed. There is an increasing awareness of both the common elements of technique used by therapists of different traditions, and the common psychological processes that may underlie response to different methods (e.g., Wachtel, 1977).

## SOCIAL AND ORGANIZATIONAL ASPECTS OF INTERVENTIONS

The psychological interventions discussed in the previous section aim to 'treat' the presenting problem in the sense of removing, or at least substantially reducing whatever abnormal behaviour or subjective distress brought the patient for treatment. This objective is not always attainable. It is not so much that there are some kinds of presenting problem that always defy treatment. Rather it is that, within the patients who present with any particular problem, there are some who are difficult to treat. Various methods have been used to identify these 'poor prognosis' patients, and biographical information has proved one of the most generally useful. There is a surprising similarity in prognostic factors across different presenting problems. In general, it is patients who have a good record of social adjustment who tend to respond better to treatment. A stable work record, a successful marital and family adjustment, and good social integration seem to be good prognostic factors in a wide variety of conditions (Phillips, 1968).

The characteristics of 'poor prognosis' patients have important implications for their psychological management. For patients who do not respond to treatment, more modest objectives need to be set. The aim has to be to help them to lead as normal lives as possible despite their problems, and to retain an appropriate level of autonomy and independence rather than becoming over-dependent on the health service and other supportive agencies. Social management of this kind is a task to which clinical psychologists have an important contribution to make, though one that draws on different areas of psychology from the kind of psychological treatments discussed in the previous section. Given that it is largely poor social adjustment that predicts, and is therefore presumably responsible for, poor response to treatment, social adjustment needs to be a central focus of such psychological management.

Some of the patients who need this approach are patients who have been hospitalized over a long period, and have acquired a variety of secondary handicaps as a result. The task is then to organize their milieu so as to reverse these handicaps and prepare them for resettlement in the community. Programmes to achieve this usually need to be set up both on the ward in which the patients live, and in the occupational unit where they go for work in activity hours.

A kind of ward programme to which psychologists have made a particular contribution is the token economy (Kazdin, 1977). This is based on the systematic application of positive reinforcements or rewards. For each patient, certain performances are identified which the programme is designed to encourage. These vary considerably depending on how institutionalized the patient has become, but improving independent self-care and increasing levels of activity and social interaction are common goals. Each time a patient achieves one of the performances on his personal programme, he is 'rewarded' by being given a token that he can subsequently exchange for goods of his choice.

Other types of ward programmes have been based on the principles of the 'therapeutic community', with particular emphasis on social and group interaction and discussion of patients' problems. There is usually an attempt to achieve democratic decision-making amongst the staff and to create a climate in which patients are accountable to the whole community for their actions (Rapoport, 1960). Other ward programmes have combined features of both systematic behavioural programmes and the therapeutic community (Shepherd, 1980). In each case a key factor in the long-term effectiveness of such programmes in ensuring the enthusiastic and sustained co-operation of the whole ward staff in the programme, and psychologists working on long-term wards need to devote a lot of time to facilitating the works of other members of the staff team.

Occupational programmes are also important in improving the social adjustment of long-term patients. Work activities can be especially important because they require patients to develop a capacity for coping with external demands that will also be needed in other social roles when they are resettled in the community. Psychologists have a particularly important role in identifying the occupational handicaps of individual patients and of ensuring that patients are provided with opportunities to remedy their deficits (Watts, 1983). Without this involvement there is a danger of occupational programmes being carried on without any clearly formulated objectives.

With modern approaches to care, the number of patients admitted to hospital for long periods has declined sharply. This has meant that it is more often possible to carry out programmes designed to improve patients' social adjustment in acute units or in community settings. Though there is no longer any need to seek to reverse the institutionalizing effects of long-term hospitalization, the objectives and methods used in the programmes are similar in other ways. A new element introduced by the community setting is the patient's family, which assumes much more importance. For many patients, improving performance in domestic and family roles is at least as important as improving their capacity for employment, and programmes to achieve this are now being developed.

The patient's family also has an important part to play in management and treatment. In many cases it will be more profitable for the psychologist to work through the patient's family rather than with the patient directly, just as a psychologist in a long-term hospital would often work through the ward staff. As with ward programmes, this might take the form of involving the family in a behavioural programme, or it might use a patient of family therapy that examines the family as a social system and change how this is affecting the 'patient' (e.g., Minuchin, 1974).

A good example of the involvement of the family in behavioural treatment is the work of Mathews *et al.* (1977) on the treatment of agoraphobia. The treatment was based on the principles of desensitization to the feared situation described earlier, but the spouse was given a particular role in working out the details of the programme, and providing help and encouragement. It is known that agoraphobics with poor marital adjustment tend to respond poorly to treatment (Hafner, 1977) and involving the spouse actively in treatment is one way of trying to overcome this. Spouses have also been involved in behavioural programmes based on reward principles for both schizophrenic (Hudson, 1975) and depressed patients (Liberman and Ruskin, 1971). In the latter, for example, very impressive results were obtained when the spouse was shown how to avoid rewarding depressive behaviour and to reward coping behaviour instead.

It has become clear, from epidemiological surveys that the number of mental health problems in the community far exceeds those that come to the psychiatric department of a hospital. Psychologists have therefore become aware of a need, if they are to move towards providing a comprehensive psychological contribution to mental health problems to operate outside this restricted context (McPherson and Sutton, 1981). However, they are also aware that the number of potential clients far exceeds anything they can hope to work with on an individual basis with their current manpower. There is thus an increasing interest in transmitting psychological skills to other professionals and agencies more directly involved in the community. Working with general practitioners is the one that has so far been most actively explored (see Chapter 13) but it seems likely that work with and through other voluntary and statutory agencies concerned with mental health is likely to become an increasingly important part of the clinical psychologist's role.

## REFERENCES


Bannister, D. (1975). *Issues and Approaches in the Psychological Therapies.* London: Wiley.

Bannister, D., and Fransella, F. (1971). *Inquiring Man: The Theory of Personal Constructs*. Harmondsworth: Penguin.

Barlow, D. H. (1981). *Behavioral Assessment of Adult Disorders.* New York: Guildford Publications.

Beck, A. T., Rush, A. J., Shaw, B. F., and Emery, G. (1979). *Cognitive Therapy of Depression.* Chichester: Wiley.

Beech, H. R., and Vaughan, M. (1978). *Behavioural Treatment of Obsessional States.* Chichester: Wiley.

Buss, A. H. (1966). *Psychopathology.* New York: Wiley.

Chapman, L. J., and Chapman, J. P. (1973). *Disordered Thought in Schizophrenia.* New York: Appleton-Century.

Di Loreto, A. O. (1971). *Comparative Psychotherapy: An Experimental Analysis.* Chicago: Aldine-Atherton.

Epstein, L. H. (1976) Psychophysiological measurement in assessment. In M. Hersen and A. S. Bellack (eds), *Behavioral Assessment: a Practical Handbook.* New York: Pergamon.

Eysenck, H. J. (1970). *The Structure of Human Personality.* London: Methuen.

Foulds, G. A. and Bedford, A. (1975). Hierarchy of classes of personal illness. *Psychological Medicine,* **5**, 181–192.

Hafner, R. J. (1977). The husbands of agoraphobic women and their influence on treatment outcome. *British Journal of Psychiatry,* **131**, 289–294.

Hudson, B. L. (1975). A behaviour modification project with chronic schizophrenics in the community. *Behaviour Research and Therapy,* **13**, 339–341.

Kazdin, A. E. (1977). *The Token Economy.* New York: Plenum.

Lewinsohn, P. M., and Shaw, D. A. (1969). Feedback about interpersonal behavior as an agent of change: A case study in the treatment of depression. *Psychotherapy and Psychosomatics,* **17**, 82–88.

Liberman, R. P. (1976). Behavior therapy for schizophrenia. In L. J. West and D. E. Flinn (eds), *Treatment of Schizophrenia: Progress and Prospects.* New York: Grune and Stratton.

Liberman, R. P., and Ruskin, D. E. (1971). Depression: A behavioural formulation. *Archives of General Psychiatry,* **24**, 515–523.

Malan, D. H. (1979). *Individual Psychotherapy and the Science of Psychodynamics.* London: Butterworth.

Mathews, A. M., Teasdale, J. D., Munby, M., Johnston, D. W., and Shaw, P. M. A. (1977). A home-based treatment program for agoraphobia. *Behavior Therapy*, **8**, 915–924.
McPherson, I., and Sutton, A. (1981). *Reconstructing Psychological Practice.* London: Croom Helm.
Meichenbaum, D. (1977). *Cognitive Behavior Modification, an Integrative Approach.* New York: Plenum.
Merluzzi, T. V., Glass, C. R., and Genest, M. (1981). *Cognitive Assessment.* New York: Guildford Publications.
Milton, F., Patwa, V. K., and Hafner, J. (1978). Confrontation vs. belief modification in persistently deluded patients. *British Journal of Medical Psychology*, **51**, 127–130.
Minuchin, S. (1974). *Families and Family Therapy.* London: Tavistock.
Mischel, W. (1968). *Personality and Assessment.* New York: Wiley.
Mitchell, K. M., Bozarth, J. D., and Krauft, C. C. (1977). A reappraisal of the therapeutic effectiveness of accurate empathy, non-possessive warmth and genuineness. In A. S. Gurman and A. M. Razin (eds), *Effective Psychotherapy: A Handbook of Research.* Oxford: Pergamon.
Novaco, R. (1975). *Anger Control: The Development and Evaluation of an Experimental Treatment.* Lexington: Heath.
Phillips, L. (1968). *Human Adaptation and its Failures.* New York: Academic Press.
Ramsay, R. W. (1979). Bereavement: A behavioral treatment of pathological grief. In P. O. Sjoden, S. Bates and W. S. Dockens (eds), *Trends in Behavior Therapy*. New York: Academic Press.
Rapoport, R. N. (1960). *Community as Doctor: New Perspectives on a Therapeutic Community.* London: Tavistock.
Rehm, L. P. (1981). *Behavior Therapy for Depression.* New York: Academic Press.
Rogers, C. R. (1951). *Client-Centered Therapy*. Boston: Houghton-Mifflin.
Sandler, J., Dare, C., and Holder, A. (1973). *The Patient and the Analyst: The Basis of the Psychoanalytic Process.* London: Allen and Unwin.
Shapiro, M. B. (1961). The single case in fundamental clinical psychological research. *British Journal of Medical Psychology*, **34**, 355–364.
Shepherd, G. W. (1980). The treatment of social difficulties in special environments. In P. Feldman and J. Orford (eds), *Psychological Problems: The Social Context.* Chichester: Wiley.
Slade, P. D. (1972). The effects of systematic desensitization on auditory hallucinations. *Behaviour Research and Therapy,* **10**, 85–91.
Szasz, T. S. (1961). *The Myth of Mental Illness.* New York: Harper and Row.
Trower, P., Bryant, B., and Argyle, M. (1978). *Social Skills and Mental Health*. London: Methuen.
Turner, S. M., Calhoun, K. S., and Adams, H. E. (1981). *Handbook of Clinical Behavior Therapy*. New York: Wiley.
Wachtel, P. L. (1977). *Psychoanalysis and Behavior Therapy: Toward an Integration.* New York: Basic Books.
Watts, F. N. (1980). Clinical judgement and clinical training. *British Journal of Medical Psychology,* **53**, 95–108.
Watts, F. N. (1983). Employment. In F. N. Watts and D. H. Bennett (eds), *Theory and Practice of Psychiatric Rehabilitation.* Wiley: Chichester.
Wolpe, J. (1969). *The Practice of Behavior Therapy*. New York: Pergamon.

The Practice of Clinical Psychology in Great Britain
Edited by A. Liddell


*Chapter 6*

# *Mentally disordered offenders*

*Ronald Blackburn*

The area of practice to be described in this chapter originates in the contact of clinical psychology with forensic psychiatry, a speciality which has been described as '. . . the application of general psychiatric principles to the problem of the mentally disordered offender at all stages of his treatment' (Home Office/Department of Health and Social Security, 1975). Broadly, then, the client group of concern is composed of those who exhibit antisocial behaviour, particularly that which threatens the welfare or safety of others, and who are also considered to be psychiatrically abnormal.

Although all countries with developed mental health services appear to make special provision for mentally disordered offenders, it is nevertheless the case that the recognition of such a group is the outcome of legal philosophy and social policy, rather than the identification of a specific kind of medical or psychological problem. One consequence of this is that the availability of services is determined as much by arbitrary administrative boundaries as by clearly defined personal need. Before the role of clinical psychologists in relation to this group is examined, the current provision of mental health services for offenders in Britain will therefore be considered.

## TREATMENT FACILITIES FOR MENTALLY DISORDERED OFFENDERS

### Health Service Facilities

The earliest statutory provision for the psychiatric treatment of offenders excused from legal punishment on the grounds of insanity is traced by McGrath (1967) to the Insane Offenders Act of 1800. This gave legal sanction for such facilities to be made available at Bethlem Hospital. Current facilities, however, are largely the result of the 1959 Mental Health Act for England and Wales (and the similar, though not identical legislation for Scotland and for Northern Ireland), which made comprehensive provision for mentally disordered offenders within the health service. The Act defines mental disorder as 'mental illness, arrested or incomplete development of mind, psychopathic disorder and any other disorder or disability of mind', and on medical evidence that an offender is suffering from such disorder, the court may discharge him, subject him to a penal sentence, impose a probation order with conditions of in-patient or out-patient treatment, or impose a hospital order requiring compulsory detention in hospital. Higher courts may additionally impose a 'restriction order', which prevents a detained patient from being discharged without the consent of the Home Secretary.

The Act also brought together under the central administration of the then Ministry of Health institutions previously built for the secure detention of 'criminal lunatics' or 'dangerous mental defectives', designating them as Special Hospitals. These are for persons who 'require treatment under conditions of special security on account of their dangerous, violent or criminal propensities'. There are now five such hospitals in Britain, these being Broadmoor, Rampton, Moss Side, and Park Lane in England, and the State Hospital in Scotland. Together, they house some 2,400 compulsorily detained patients, four-fifths of them male. About 70 per cent have committed serious crimes such as murder, arson, or sexual assault, but the hospitals also admit convicted prisoners who become psychiatrically disordered in prison, and psychiatric patients who exhibit violent behaviour in other hospitals.

The Special Hospitals admit only a small proportion of mentally disordered offenders, who in turn represent only a small minority of all psychiatric patients or all offenders. For example, of the 197,188 admissions to psychiatric hospitals in 1973, 27,331 came from the courts, penal establishments, or the police. In that year, the Special Hospitals admitted 371 patients (Home Office/Department of Health and Social Security, 1975). Psychiatric disposals also accounted for less than a half of one per cent of the three-quarters of a million convictions for offences other than motoring offences. The majority of mentally disordered offenders, then, are dealt with in open psychiatric hospitals, and not under special treatment conditions.

On the other hand, it has been estimated that between 1 per cent and 2 per cent of the prison population fall within the statutory definition of mental disorder (Royal College of Psychiatrists, 1980), while as many as a third of convicted prisoners have some history of psychiatric disability (Gunn, 1977). Although the penal system has a long established medical service, and some attempts are made to cater for psychiatric problems within penal establishments (including the setting up of a psychiatric prison for selected male offenders at Grendon Underwood in 1962), there appears to be a consensus that many offenders who currently receive prison sentences would be better dealt with by the mental health services.

The passing of the Mental Health Act coincided with the emergence of the liberalized 'open door' policy of psychiatric hospital treatment, one result of which has been that there are now relatively few health service facilities for patients whose behaviour warrants some degree of secure containment, but at a level less than that of the maximum security afforded by the Special Hospitals.

The Butler Committee (Home Office/Department of Health and Social Security, 1975) identified a need for such facilities, and recommended the setting up of Regional Secure Units in England and Wales. To date, one has been built, three 'interim' secure units are in operation, and planning is at an advanced stage for a further eight units. The Royal College of Psychiatrists (1980) has in addition proposed that there should be smaller and more local treatment facilities offering security (by which is meant not only physical containment, but also a high staff–patient ratio), although their concern is for psychiatric patients whose violent behaviour poses problems of nursing management, and those regarded as 'social inadequates', categories which may include but are not confined to offenders.

Whether or not security conditions are involved, this provision of health service facilities for offenders is commonly regarded as the domain of forensic psychiatry. The use of this term to denote specialized treatment is, however, misleading. Both etymologically and in established usage, the adjective 'forensic' applies to argument within a legal setting, and forensic experts, whatever their discipline, are those who examine and present evidence to the court in relation to a particular case (Haward, 1976). The adjective does not, therefore, describe an area of clinical skill or scientific knowledge but rather the application of such knowledge in a specific judicial context. Only when a psychiatrist assesses and presents evidence on the mental state of a person before the court can he properly he said to be exercising a forensic function.

The issue is not simply one of semantic impropriety, since to extend the description 'forensic' to therapeutic activities implies that the clinician is a specialist treating something not dealt with by his 'non-forensic' colleagues. There is evidence that criminal populations are likely to contain large numbers of individuals suffering from personality disorder, alcohol addiction, and mental retardation, and that crimes of violence, sexual offences, and drug offences are more likely to be associated with psychiatric disturbance than are property offences (Gunn, 1977). However, with the possible exception of psychopathic (or antisocial) personality, there is no category of psychiatric disorder which is unique to the mentally disordered offender. Apart from the provision of evidence to the court, then, there is little in the way of the therapeutic goals or methods which forensic psychiatry does not share with general psychiatry. It is the mental disorder of the mentally disordered offender, not his offending behaviour, which determines placement in the mental health system. The same is no less true of those treated in Special Hospitals or secure units. Mental disorder, not dangerousness, is the target of medical treatment.

This is not to say that antisocial behaviour in general, or dangerous behaviour in particular, is an incidental consideration. But implicit in the identification of the mentally disordered offender is the assumption that his mental disorder is the cause of the offending behaviour, and that amelioration of the disorder is a precondition for removing antisocial tendencies. As will be argued later, this is frequently a tenuous assumption which may lead to inappropriate treatment goals.

**Psychological Services for Offenders**

The kind of psychological services available to offenders is determined to a large extent by administrative factors. Most clinical psychologists working with psychiatric patients or the mentally handicapped probably work from time to time with clients referred through the courts. Services to juvenile offenders are also available from educational psychologists. However, a recent survey indicates that only about 40 clinical psychologists working within the National Health Service currently have regular commitments to offenders, and this represents under 4 per cent of national manpower. Almost half of these work in Special Hospitals or secure units, and receive most of their referrals through forensic psychiatrists. The remainder are based in Area Psychology Departments, penal establishments, or local authority centres, and receive referrals directly from the courts, probation officers, or the prisons, as well as from medical sources. Not all clients, then, will have been identified as mentally disordered in the statutory sense, although most probably have.

Prison psychologists form an administratively separate group in England and Wales (but not in Scotland or Northern Ireland, where services to the prisons are available through clinical psychologists), and have somewhat different professional aims from those of clinical or educational psychologists. Although their functions are broadly rehabilitative, they are numerically small relative to the prison population, and they do not aim to provide individual services for more than a small proportion of prisoners. In 1976, Twiselton noted that there were 80 prison psychologists in post, of whom 10 were either qualified or receiving training in clinical psychology, but that the general strategy of the service was to concentrate on the '. . . design, development and evaluation aspects of the organisation, its staff, and its procedures'.

As well as those concerned with offenders, there is a number of psychologists investigating behaviour within the legal system, such as the decision-making of juries, or witness testimony, and the growth of these converging interests was reflected by the setting up of the Division of Criminological and Legal Psychology within the British Psychological Society in 1977. However, the term forensic psychologist has been subject to the same loose usage as that of forensic psychiatrist. Although the courts in Britain have been slower than those in the United States to acknowledge behavioural scientists as expert witnesses, clinical and educational psychologists may be required to present evidence to the court on the psychological characteristics of an accused person. Also, a few psychologists have achieved recognition as expert witnesses, and have been called to present opinions based on tests or experiments regarding such matters as the mental state or functioning of the accused, or the probability of particular acts occurring or being witnessed (Haward, 1969). This function also extends to civil cases, such as obscenity trials or mercantile disputes involving customer behaviour. While Haward (1969) notes that clinical psychologists are well placed to develop this role because of their training in both applied and experimental psychology, clinical matters form only a part of the work of the forensic psychologist. Moreover, the psychologist appearing as an expert witness is serving the purposes of the court. This is quite different from providing therapeutic services for an offender, or studying behaviour in legal settings.

It is therefore preferable to confine the term forensic psychologist to those who collect and present evidence for a specific judicial purpose. At the present time, clinical psychologists working with offenders do not typically exercise this function. However, it is contrary to the Rule of Hearsay for data from a psychologist's examination to be incorporated into medical testimony (Ward, 1978), and psychologists are therefore professionally bound to draw attention to the independence and admissibility of their evidence in criminal trials.

## CLINICAL PSYCHOLOGY AND THE MENTALLY DISORDERED OFFENDER

### Therapeutic Goals and Strategies

In terms of training and role, there is little difference between the work of clinical psychologists who work with offenders and that of psychologists working in other parts of the health service. Similarly, there is overlap with the work of applied psychologists in penal or educational settings. However, the more distinctive features of this work are seen in security settings catering for 'dangerous' patients, most of whom will have committed aggressive or sexual crimes. The remainder of the chapter will focus on work in this context.

It was pointed out earlier that placement of the mentally disordered offender in the health service implies a need for medical treatment of the disorder. This is justifiable to the extent that a potentially treatable mental disorder has been identified, and a link between the disorder and the offending behaviour established. But it is doubtful whether either of these conditions is universally met. Those identified as mentally disordered offenders form a very heterogeneous group, both in terms of disorder and offending behaviour, and this applies equally to those singled out as dangerous. For example, while the largest subgroup consists of those categorized as suffering from Mental Illness in terms of the Mental Health Act, about a third of those admitted to Special Hospitals fall in the statutory category of Psychopathic Disorder, and a quarter in the categories of Subnormality or Severe Subnormality. Whatever the arguments about the appropriateness of the 'mental illness' metaphor, it is in practice the case that pharmacological or other medical treatment is likely to offer the best strategy for treating psychotic disorder (which accounts for most of the Mental Illness category). This cannot be said for the remaining categories, whose 'treatability' by medical means is doubtful. Furthermore, apart from the absence of any general causal relationship between psychiatric disorder and crime, the relation for any given individual is frequently obscure. It may appear reasonable, for example, to attribute to mental illness the behaviour of someone who attacks the subject of persecutory delusions. But sexual assault by a mentally retarded person is in no way explained by low intelligence. Still more problematic is the case where a 'personality disorder' is inferred from a history of violent sex crimes. For many identified as mentally disordered offenders, then, the attribution of deviant behaviour to a mental disorder is of little help either as explanation or in indicating appropriate treatment goals.

For these reasons, psychologists working in this area regard the antisocial behaviour of such offenders as the appropriate target of therapeutic intervention (British Psychological Society, 1973: Black, 1976). It is the variables of which this behaviour is a function which need to be dealt with, and while these may include identifiable states of 'illness', a much broader range of psychological and social problems has to be considered. These include lack of social, educational, or occupational skills, unusual personal attributes such as excessive shyness or aggressiveness, deviant values or attitudes to oneself or others, and inappropriate ways of reacting to stresses or particular social interactions. It is attention to variables such as these, rather than to a supposed disorder 'underlying' them, which is seen as affording the most appropriate strategy for reducing the likelihood of further dangerous behaviour. Although psychologists differ in the extent to which they attach significance to particular kinds of problem, approaches in this area have been influenced primarily by behavioural methods of treatment, in which the focus is on relatively specific problems, and the promotion of more appropriate behaviour through the provision of active learning experiences. In these terms, treatment refers to the social analogue of remedial education rather than to the elimination of disease.

It would, however, be an oversimplification to assume a clear dichotomy between those who need medical treatment and those who require rehabilitation through non-medical procedures. In our present state of knowledge, all therapeutic measures for dealing with dangerous offenders are tentative, and there are few problems for which there is a single prescribed treatment. Attempts to change the deviant behaviour of sex offenders, for example, have included both psychological and pharmacological methods. Moreover, the contribution of the psychologist is likely to vary both for different patients and for differing stages of a patient's treatment, as when the facilitation of ward management of an acute psychotic patient through behavioural training supplements drug treatment and nursing care. This means that the psychologist must be in a position to identify when his professional skills may (or may not) be of benefit to the patient, either directly, or indirectly through collaboration with other treatment staff. This can be accomplished only through membership of a multidisciplinary psychiatric team.

**Treatment, Assessment, and Research**

Within the Special Hospitals, the first psychology departments were set up at Rampton in 1954, and at Broadmoor in 1959. The role of psychologists working in secure settings of this kind has undergone the same kind of changes which have characterized clinical psychology more generally in recent years.

Where, for example, in 1967 the medical superintendent of Broadmoor saw the contribution of psychologists as primarily research and investigation of the individual patient (McGrath, 1967), the Royal College of Psychiatrists (1980) envisages the role of clinical psychologists in secure units as involving 'therapy, evaluation and teaching of in-patients and out-patients', and considers it unlikely that such units can function properly without this contribution. There has therefore been a shift of emphasis from the provision of diagnostic and prognostic information based on psychological tests to a more active involvement in treatment and rehabilitation.

This is not to say that assessment and research have ceased to be significant components of the role of psychologists in this area. The decision as to when a dangerous patient is suitable for release is a central clinical function of the work of Special Hospitals' staff, and this demands the use of objective predictors and the reliable assessment of psychological change (Black, 1981). At the same time, the development of effective assessment and therapeutic procedures is only possible through systematic evaluation of their utility. Research into the psychology of antisocial behaviour, the predictive utility of assessment devices, and the outcome of treatment procedures has, in fact, increased steadily in recent years, and accounts for almost half of all research within the Special Hospitals. Nevertheless, it is in the area of treatment methods that the most significant developments are taking place.

Patients in Special Hospitals are effectively subject to indeterminate detention, but the hospitals share with penal institutions the problem of providing realistic rehabilitation programmes within the confines of an institution. While it has been claimed that the artificiality of such environments is one reason why attempts to rehabilitate offenders have not been very successful, a survey of recent psychological approaches to the treatment of offenders suggests that this may be an unduly pessimistic view, and that some programmes in penal institutions can have a significant impact on subsequent behaviour outside the institution (Blackburn, 1980). This appears to be particularly the case with methods which focus on providing the offender with skills which promote more effective adaptation in the community, not only the educational achievement-related or vocational skills required for urban living, but in particular the social skills involved in establishing effective interpersonal relationships. A viewpoint which has recently gained ground among psychologists is, in fact, that many antisocial acts occur not because of perverse or abnormal needs or dispositions, but because the offender lacks appropriate skills for attaining his ends in more acceptable ways. This may be equally true of many aggressive and sexual offenders. Rape and child molestation, for example, are not uncommonly the acts of men who lack the basic skills of interpersonal communication required to promote effective relationships with an adult female. A 'social skills training' approach to the treatment of such offenders has consequently been a significant recent development in this area.

Such an approach is illustrated by the work of Howells (1976) with aggressive offenders. Research at Broadmoor has indicated that not all serious assaults are committed by habitually violent offenders, and that some acts of extreme aggression, such as murder, are perpetrated by individuals who are more typically mild-mannered and 'overcontrolled' (Blackburn, 1971). These individuals appear to have strong inhibitions against behaving aggressively, and their offences seem to represent the unusual expression of intense anger in the face of extreme or accumulated provocation. A lack of appropriate self-assertion or acceptable ways of expressing anger may therefore be a significant contributor to the development of interpersonal frustration and conflict experienced by these individuals. Howells suggests that training in assertiveness and in coping directly with anger-arousing situations rather than avoiding them may benefit such patients. He describes a training programme in which an analysis is made of the patient's behaviour in a simulated anger-provoking situation (role-play). The patient is given feedback of his behaviour from a videotaped recording, and by means of demonstration (modelling), discussion, and praise for appropriate behaviour, learns alternative modes of responding. In addition to illustrating how this approach was used to teach assertiveness to a murderer who typically avoided making appropriate reactions to annoyance, Howells also showed its applicability to a persistently aggressive offender. In this case, analysis of typical behaviour sequences revealed the patient's tendency to maximize conflict in a social encounter by arguing, criticizing, and finally threatening violence, and ways of behaving which would avoid this sequence were taught through role-play. Howells (1981) suggests that training of this kind needs to include the patient's awareness of his emotional state, and also how he interprets the behaviour of others. The long-term effects of this approach, however, have yet to be evaluated.

A similar procedure has been applied to the behaviour deficits of sex offenders. Crawford (1978) describes a programme of group training for patients with a history of sexual assaults. The patients' typical social reactions were first assessed by means of questionnaires and self-ratings of social anxiety, and through observations of role-play in a number of social interactions. These procedures were used to identify individual problems and to provide a baseline against which to assess change. Treatment consisted of weekly sessions with a male and female therapist, and involved role-play, videotaped feedback, and discussion. Behaviour dealt with progressed from non-verbal responses such as posture and eye-contact, to vocalization, conversational techniques, and finally to behaviour in common social situations. Patients were also encouraged to attend to appropriate behaviour at hospital social functions, such as dances. After four months of this training, significant improvements in social functioning were demonstrated in comparison with a similar group for whom treatment was deferred.

A more traditional behavioural approach to the treatment of sexual deviation has been to focus directly on the elimination of deviant sexual interests. Electrical and chemical aversion treatments based on conditioning principles have been available for some time, but apart from a limited success rate, objections to their use have been made on both aesthetic and ethical grounds.

An alternative approach to the treatment of sex offenders through the use of self-control methods is described by Lee-Evans (1978). In behavioural terms, this refers to the use by the individual of responses which control the deviant behaviour, either by competing with it, for example, by avoiding children's television in the case of a pedophile, or suppressing it through imagining unpleasant consequences. The development of self-controlling responses is taught through a combination of methods which involve becoming aware of the environmental conditions which lead to deviant thoughts and sexual arousal, the daily recording by the patient of when and how these occur, and through encouragement to use self-praise when controlling responses are effective, or criticism when they are not. Lee-Evans points to the role of masturbatory fantasies in maintaining sexual interests, and describes attempts to eliminate these through self-control. At the same time, 'shaping' methods employing pictorial stimuli were used to generate acceptable alternative heterosexual fantasies.

These complementary approaches to the treatment of sex offenders have not, as yet, been used extensively, and several problems surrounding their use remain. In social skills training, for example, the kind of behaviour learned needs to be appropriate to the patient's own sociocultural setting, but what is most acceptable is not always clear. There is also the problem of generalizing effects from the closed institution to the natural environment outside. Self-control methods have the potential for facilitating generalization by providing the patient with a means of manipulating his own environment. But a security hospital offers limited opportunities for natural practice of newly acquired behaviour or for assessing the effectiveness of training. It is unlikely that this can be overcome except through the continuation of therapy after discharge from hospital.

It would also be unduly simplistic to see the problems of sex offenders exclusively in terms of deviant sexual interest and lack of heterosexual skills. Crawford (1979) notes that sex offenders tend to show a variety of social and sexual problems which demand comprehensive therapeutic attention. Anxiety about heterosexual behaviour, for example, is a common problem in this group. Crawford describes the use of a sex education programme which had the effect of reducing anxiety and increasing subjective confidence in sexual performance.

These examples of developments in the psychological treatment of dangerous offenders involve the psychologist directly functioning as a behaviour analyst and modifier. However, the psychologist's role in relation to the psychiatric team is not confined to that of a specialist therapist to whom selected patients are referred. Indeed, in view of the small number of clinical psychologists currently available in this area, an effective deployment of their time may involve an emphasis on the teaching of behaviour change methods to other clinical staff rather than on individual treatment. This role has been developed in the context of a multidisciplinary rehabilitation team in an 'interim' regional secure unit (Reid *et al.*, 1980). The aim of the team is to provide patients with independent living skills, using a multifaceted behavioural approach to treatment. The psychologist spends some of the time carrying out social skills training in conjunction with other staff, and may also provide relaxation training for patients who experience tension or social anxiety. However, teaching selected nursing staff to execute behaviour change procedures is seen as a major function. While the psychologist is involved in the design of individual behaviour modification programmes, these are carried out by nurse therapists, and members of the patient's family may also be involved.

An essential requirement for the successful application of the kind of treatment methods discussed is the availability of adequate assessment procedures for identifying problems and evaluating change. Psychiatric diagnostic classification indicates a patient's problems in only very gross terms, and hence is of little value in planning individual psychological treatment. While traditional psychological tests may supply clinically relevant information on such matters as achievement-related skills, intellectual deterioration or the presence of organic brain disorder, routine diagnostic testing of dangerous offenders is similarly unlikely to make sufficient contribution to clinical decision-making to be justified.

Tests measuring broad personality traits such as aggressiveness, sociability, or anxiety-proneness may indicate how a person behaves in general, but do not yield very reliable information about the kinds of behaviour a person shows in particular situations. Davis (1974), for example, showed that the scales of a personality test, the SHAPS (Special Hospitals' Assessment of Personality and Socialization: Blackburn, 1974), were able to predict the aggressive and sociable behaviour of patients in a Rampton ward, as observed directly and as rated by nursing staff, but the level of prediction was not sufficiently high to predict accurately the hospital behaviour of individual patients. On the other hand, research with this test (Blackburn, 1975; 1979) has indicated that four distinct personality patterns can be identified among dangerous offenders, and that these have some relationship with such characteristics as different levels of nervous system activity, vividness of imagery, and history of violent crime. This work has indicated that the controversial concept of the psychopath can be given relatively precise meaning when used as a description of personality. While tests of this kind are currently most useful as research tools or for global screening decisions, it is conceivable that they may turn out to have predictive value in clinical practice. We know very little, for example, about the extent to which generalized attributes of the individual determine his responsiveness to different kinds of therapeutic approach. In this context, Lee-Evans (1978) suggests that Internal–External Locus of Control, a personality dimension related to beliefs about the degree of personal control over events, may indicate which patients are more likely to respond to self-control training.

The assessment procedures currently regarded as most useful in this area are those which focus on specific psychological characteristics likely to be relevant to behaviourally oriented treatments. Typically, these are individualized tests or *ad hoc* self or observer ratings rather than traditional standardized tests.

Howells has employed the Repertory Grid Test to assess the personal meaning of significant events or people to patients, and illustrates its use in the case of a poisoner (Howells, 1978). A similar procedure, the Semantic Differential, has been used to evaluate the relative attractiveness of different sexual stimuli to sex offenders (Lee-Evans, 1978). Self-ratings of the degree of social anxiety in particular situations, structured ward observations of specific communication, occupational and domestic skills, and observations of behaviour in role-play situations are other examples of assessment methods which have been used to identify problem behaviour or skill deficits, and which provide a baseline against which to monitor the progress of treatment programmes.

Particular attention has been directed at the problem of assessing deviant sexual interest. Verbal reports of sexual fantasies, or ratings of the attractiveness of sexual stimuli are under voluntary control, and hence fakeable, and are not related in any simple fashion to sexual arousal. Attempts at objective measurement of sexual arousal to relevant stimuli presented on slides or film have employed penile plethysmography, which involves recording changes in the volume of the penis by means of a thin, mercury-filled loop. Changes in penile volume, however, are also under voluntary control, for example, through avoiding attending to the stimulus. Cliffe (1977) has described an objective laboratory procedure in which the relative rates of responding to two different levers producing different visual sexual stimuli can yield quantifiable information regarding sexual preference. Again, however, responding is subject to voluntary control.

Faking is an issue only if a patient is suspected of not being fully co-operative, and in the context of a trusting therapeutic relationship both verbal and physiological measures are of value in monitoring the progress of treatment. Nevertheless, the concern to eliminate faking arises because of the need to predict the likelihood of an offender committing further dangerous offences, a major consideration in the psychiatric decision to discharge a patient from secure detention. The evidence to date indicates that our capacity to predict dangerousness is inadequate, and neither intuitive clinical judgement, actuarial indices derived from previous history, nor psychological tests have been shown to be able to separate the potentially dangerous offender from the non-dangerous (Hinton, 1983). The typical error is over-prediction of dangerousness, in that many who are thought likely to commit further violent crimes will not in fact do so. One problem is that repetition of a dangerous crime is a relatively rare event, and prediction under these conditions demands decision-making aids of a much higher precision than are currently available. Another dificulty is that dangerous crimes are frequently as much a product of temporary mood disturbance, alcohol intoxication, or situational factors as of identifiable personal characteristics. Nevertheless, dangerousness predictions have to be made, and it is appropriate that psychological research should be directed at improving them. Black (1977) has reported a five-year follow-up of patients released from Broadmoor, and found that personality test data showed some relationship to further violent offences, although past history of dangerous behaviour was the best single predictor. Combining data of this sort by statistical means may produce improved criteria. However, it is probable that the most practical strategy is to specify in advance the identifiable psychological changes which need to take place for dangerous behaviour to be less likely, and to make these the goals of therapeutic intervention.

**Some Problems of Clinical Work in Secure Settings**

It has already been noted that high security institutions impose limits on the implementation of behavioural treatment programmes, and that reliance often has to be placed on indirect methods or simulation of natural conditions in evaluating psychological change. Apart from these constraints on professional practice, clinical psychologists share with other staff problems arising from the social climate of an institution which must maintain a balance between the dual functions of protecting the public from the patient and providing treatment which is in the best interests of individual patients.

This balance can sometimes break down, and in the absence of clearly defined and optimistic clinical policies, security and containment may become the dominant goal of the institution and of significant sections of its staff (Department of Health and Social Security, 1980). Under such conditions, innovative therapeutic strategies engender conflict and compromise. In an effort to establish his therapeutic credentials, it is all too easy for the psychologist to become involved in patient management procedures which may serve the purposes of institutional control, but which may have little to do with the problems which brought the patient to the institution in the first place. To ensure effective delivery of psychological services, it is essential for the psychologist to have a role in institutional management and in defining overall clinical policies.

There are also ethical issues surrounding the treatment of patients who have been hospitalized involuntarily and for an indeterminate period. Any attempt to reduce the likelihood of dangerous behaviour inevitably involves the psychologist in the role of agent of social control, yet for both ethical and practical reasons, he can offer his services only to those who are willing to take advantage of them. In any treatment setting, the therapist must capitalize on the variety of reasons a client has for behaviour change. In the context of a security hospital or unit, however, release is typically contingent on such change. The problem, then, is to ensure therapeutic compliance which is motivated by a desire for lasting change rather than simply release from detention.

## REFERENCES

Black, D. A. (1976). Review of the Butler Report on mentally abnormal offenders. *Bulletin of The British Psychological Society,* **29**, 130–139.

Black, D. A. (1977). A five-year follow up study of male patients discharged from Broadmoor. *Bulletin of The British Psychological Society,* **30**, 150 (Abstract).

Black, D. A. (1981). History, development and policy of the department. *Bulletin of The*

*British Psychological Society,* **34**, 35 (Abstract).
Blackburn, R. (1971). Personality types among abnormal homicides. *British Journal of Criminology,* **11**, 14–31.
Blackburn, R. (1974). Development and validation of scales to measure hostility and aggression. *Special Hospitals Research Reports, No. 12.* London: Special Hospitals Research Unit.
Blackburn, R. (1975). An empirical classification of psychopathic personality. *British Journal of Psychiatry,* **127**, 456–460.
Blackburn, R. (1979) Cortical and autonomic arousal in primary and secondary psychopaths. *Psychophysiology,* **16**, 143–150.
Blackburn, R. (1980). Still not working? A look at recent outcomes in offender rehabilitation. Paper presented at the Scottish Branch of The British Psychological Society Conference on 'Deviance', University of Stirling.
British Psychological Society (1973). Memorandum of evidence to the Butler Committee on the law relating to the mentally abnormal offender. *Bulletin of The British Psychological Society,* **26**, 331–342.
Cliffe, M. J. (1977). On an empirical calculus of reinforcement magnitude. *Archives of Sexual Behaviour,* **6**, 237–243.
Crawford, D. A. (1978). A social skills training programme with sex offenders. In J. Gunn (ed.), *Sex Offenders: A Symposium*. London: Special Hospitals Research Unit.
Crawford, D. A. (1979). Modification of deviant sexual behaviour: The need for a comprehensive approach. *British Journal of Medical Psychology,* **52**, 151–156.
Davis, H. M. (1974). Psychometric prediction of institutional adjustment. *British Journal of Social and Clinical Psychology,* **13**, 269–276.
Department of Health and Social Security (1980). *Report on the Review of Rampton Hospital.* London: HMSO.
Gunn, J. (1977). Criminal behaviour and mental disorder. *British Journal of Psychiatry,* **130**, 317–329.
Haward, L. R. C. (1969). The role of the psychologist in English Criminal Law. *Journal of Forensic Psychology,* **1**, 11–22.
Haward, L. R. C. (1976). Correspondence. *Bulletin of The British Psychological Society,* **29**, 86–87.
Hinton, J. (1983). *Dangerousness: Problems of Assessment and Prediction.* London: Allen & Unwin.
Home Office/Department of Health and Social Security (1975). *Report of the Committee on Abnormal Offenders.* London: HMSO.
Howells, K. (1976). Interpersonal aggression. *International Journal of Criminology and Penology,* **4**, 319–330.
Howells, K. (1978). The meaning of poisoning to a person diagnosed as a psychopath. *Medicine Science and The Law,* **18**, 179–184.
Howells, K. (1981). Developments in clinical approaches to the modification of violence. *Bulletin of The British Psychological Society,* **34**, 35–36 (Abstract).
Lee-Evans, J. M. (1978). The potential of self-control training procedures in the treatment of sex offenders. In J. Gunn (ed.), *Sex Offenders: A Symposium*. London: Special Hospitals Research Unit.
McGrath, P. G. (1967). The offender as an in-patient. *Royal Society Health Journal,* **87**, 329–331.
Reid, A., Lea, J., and Wallace, D. (1980). Rehabilitation on Elton Ward, an interim regional secure unit: A description of the unit after three and a half years. Unpublished manuscript, Department of Psychology, Prestwich Hospital, Manchester.
Royal College of Psychiatrists (1980). *Secure Facilities for Psychiatric Patients: A Comprehensive Policy*. London: Royal College of Psychiatrists.
Twiselton, G. (1976). Correspondence. *Bulletin of The British Psychological Society,* **29**, 311–312.

Ward, E. S. (1978). On a point of evidence. *Bulletin of The British Psychological Society*, **31**, 8–10.

The Practice of Clinical Psychology in Great Britain
Edited by A. Liddell


*Chapter 7*

# *Mental Handicap*

*Janet Carr*

Over the last thirty years it has become increasingly clear that mental handicap is not primarily a medical problem, and the work of psychologists has been of growing importance in the field. While many forms of severe mental handicap can be traced back to some physical cause (brain damage, chromosomal anomalies, etc.) there are few that are amenable to medical treatment. Treatment consists for the most part in providing the optimal conditions in which the mentally handicapped person can develop, to the fullest possible extent, the abilities that he has, and the most effective approaches are educational, social, and behavioural. The psychologist has a major role to play, in assessment, in devising and implementing programmes to promote learning and overcome behaviour problems, in management, and in teaching other professionals, parents, and caretakers.

This chapter will concentrate on work with the severely mentally handicapped since work with the mildly handicapped is more akin to that with people of normal intelligence.

## ASSESSMENT

Assessment was at one time the main preoccupation of the clinical psychologist, and the intelligence test constituted most of what he or she had to offer the mentally handicapped. Mental testing is out of vogue at present but assessment is still of major importance in this field (Mittler, 1973). The purposes of it are:

1. To establish the present level of functioning of the individual: 'most children placed in JTCs are undoubtedly severely subnormal' (Mittler, 1973) but mistakes can still happen. A difficult or unresponsive child may be wrongly regarded as severely subnormal and if it can be established by testing that he is functioning at a higher level than appeared, this can be crucial in reorienting the ideas of those about to despatch him to an ESN(S) school. Where a child or adult is handicapped it is important to assess as

clearly as possible the degree of his handicap, so that appropriate decisions can be taken regarding the type of treatment and training likely to benefit him most. For example, although severely and moderately handicapped children (IQ 20–50) can benefit from a nursery-school type environment (Lyle, 1960; Tizard, 1960) this seems to be less effective for the profoundly handicapped (IQ less than 20) for whom a different regime should be sought (Stephen and Robertson, 1970).

2. As a preliminary to treatment. Through a careful assessment it should be possible to determine the individual's particular strengths and weaknesses, suggesting which treatment approach is likely to be most useful; those behaviours and abilities that he has which need to be strengthened or developed, those which are absent and need to be established, and those which are present but need to be discouraged; and to establish the priorities for treatment. 'Assessment is the crucial first stage as it tells us . . . where to start' (Williams, 1980).

3. To monitor the effects of treatment. Once treatment is under way the person should periodically be reassessed in order to see whether the treatment is having the intended effect, and whether therefore it should be continued or revised (Kazdin, 1975).

The clinical psychologist may use many different approaches to assessment in mental handicap: standardized tests, rating scales, observational methods; information from others; and experimental approaches.

**Standardized Assessment Instruments**

The use of standardized intelligence and developmental tests is often seen as inappropriate for the severely mentally handicapped since few of the tests are standardized on this population; and, since for this group scores may be many standard deviations below the mean score for their age, the resulting IQs are distorted and cannot be related to the IQs gained by the normal population (Shakespeare, 1970). Nevertheless, especially perhaps for children, the tests offer a useful first step in providing a fairly wide-ranging series of tasks in which their competence in, for example, the use of speech and comprehension of language, hand–eye co-ordination, spatial and number skills can be observed. In addition although the age related IQs (IQ = MA/CA × 100) resulting from these tests are not comparable with conventional IQs in the normal population they may yet give useful information on the child's position within the mentally handicapped population, and a baseline from which future development may be measured. (This latter may be especially important in those cases where the child is suspected of having a degenerative condition.) Some psychologists prefer to report mental ages rather than IQs (Shakespeare, 1970), though this practice has the disadvantage of making it difficult to compare progress over time.

For testing mentally handicapped adults the WAIS (Wechsler Adult Intelligence Scale) or the British Ability Scales are most often used. For children the tests most commonly used are, first, for the youngest and most severely mentally handicapped, the infant development scales, usually either the Griffiths (Griffiths, 1954, Bayley, 1969) or Sheridan (Sheridan, 1968). In these the items start with those suitable for babies of a few days old, which ensures that even the most profoundly handicapped child is likely to be able to demonstrate his ability in some area. For the older and more competent children the Merrill-Palmer Scale (Stutsman, 1931) and the Minnesota Pre-School Scale are suitable for those with a mental age over 18 months. All these tests contain many non-verbal items which makes them especially useful for those without speech, as are also the English Picture Vocabulary Test (Brimer and Dunn, 1962) in which the child has to identify one of four pictures ('show me the . . .') and the Leiter Scale (Leiter International Performance Scale, published by C. N. Stoelting) originally developed for deaf children.

The Wechsler Intelligence Scale for Children (WISC) and the Wechsler Preschool and Primary Scale of Intelligence (WPPSI) which are widely used with normal young children, are of value only with the older and moderately or mildly handicapped children and are almost always too advanced to be used with the severely mentally handicapped.

Two rather different kinds of assessment instrument are the Sensori-Motor Scale of Piaget (Woodward, 1959) and the Behaviour Assessment Battery (Kiernan and Jones, 1977). The Sensori-Motor Scale, going up to 18 months of mental age, may be useful with a child who resists normal testing in that it does not require a set testing routine or standard test objects but may be carried out using any toy or object that the child is interested in. Although the scale classifies children's responses rather crudely, into six 'stages' between birth and 18 months, results have been found to correlate quite highly (0.54 – 0.76) with assessment of daily living skills (Garfield and Shakespeare, 1964) and, in young children with Down's syndrome, with the results of testing on the Bayley Scales (Carr, 1971). The BAB is of particular value in the assessment of the profoundly mentally handicapped, providing a broad coverage of potential skills — communication, play, problem-solving, self-help — and to a lesser extent, of emotional and social behaviour. The items are criterion-referenced and the information gained can lead directly to teaching programmes, although these may be altered and adapted as teaching proceeds.

## Rating Scales

The modern clinical psychologist is reluctant to describe any individual as 'untestable' (Berger and Yule, 1972) but, especially with the profoundly handicapped, there will be occasions when a child or adult is very difficult to test, or for some other reason seems to have given an inadequate account of himself in the test. In this case one of the published rating scales, either the Vineland (Doll, 1953) or the Gunzberg Progress Assessment Charts (Gunzberg, 1963) may be used. In these the information on what the child or adult can or cannot do is taken from his parents or someone who knows him well, and recorded according to the normal developmental sequence. The Vineland contains few items at each age level and so is not very suitable for measuring the (slow) progress of a severely mentally handicapped person. Nevertheless, it has been found to correlate well with other assessment measures, particularly in adults (Hurst, 1962; Johnson, 1970). The PAC compares ability levels in different areas — self-help, communication, socialization, and occupation — and although not a standardized measure, is widely used by nursing staff to identify areas in which help should be given.

**Observational Methods**

Observation may be used to get data on a whole range of an individual's behaviour, or may be focused on one or two specific behaviours. Examples of the first might be observations of how a child interacts with other children, or of how he responds to toys, of an adult's sexual behaviour, or, for either age group, of competence in self-help skills such as feeding, washing, dressing, and toileting. These observations may be made not only by the psychologist but also by others in the multidisciplinary team — teachers, nurses, occupational therapists, speech therapists, doctors — and the psychologist may then have the task of co-ordinating these observations into the assessment of the individual. The information gained from these observations will help to fill out the general picture, to show what skills the individual already has, what he needs to learn and where to start teaching him. More specific kinds of behaviour that may be systematically observed are, for example, self-injurious behaviour, or use of words or speech sounds. This kind of observation will often be used as a preliminary to treatment to gain a clear picture of the behaviour of interest, and so that further measures taken during or after treatment will show whether or not this is effective. The observations must then be recorded, and there are a number of different approaches to the recording of observational data that may be used (Yule, 1980). Recent evidence (Murphy and Goodall, 1980) has shown that interval recording (showing simply whether or not a behaviour occurred in a given interval, regardless of its frequency) gives estimates of the frequency of the behaviour which are at variance with the true frequency. Time-sampling, however (recording whether or not the behaviour occurred at specific moments, such as the last two seconds of a given interval), gives estimates that are much nearer to the true frequency, and this is especially important where before-and-after estimates are required (for example, before and after treatment). In addition the apparently simple procedure of interval sampling can be time-consuming and wearing (Carr, 1980a) and the apparently more rigorous time-sampling can be found to be less effort. Nevertheless, time sampling is a complex procedure and there are many occasions for which the simpler methods of event or duration recording are quite adequate.

Wherever possible observations are made independently but simultaneously by two or more observers, in order to gain a measure of the reliability of the observations. When such checks are not made even conscientious observers become careless (Reid, 1970) and the data may be misleading. Validity of the observations — whether what is reported is what actually happened — is obviously crucial (Wahler and Leske, 1973) but, except in elaborately designed experimental set-ups, very hard to ensure.

During the observation periods information may be obtained not only on the individual's skills and behaviours but also on what he likes and enjoys, which may suggest possible reinforcers to be used in teaching. Parents, or others who know him well, often also provide good information on his preferences, and these may then be tried out to test their efficacy as reinforcers. Where little is known about his preferences, or where it seems desirable to look for extra reinforcers so that a variety may be used in teaching (Kiernan, 1974), these are deliberately explored. All sorts of conventional and unconventional pleasures — noise makers, flashing lights and other sensory stimuli, fruit, cheese, crisps, soft drinks — may be tried systematically, offering the individual a choice and seeing which he consistently selects. There is some evidence that profoundly handicapped children, who respond to little else, may be reinforced by vibration (Murphy, 1982). These items too may then be tested to see whether the child not only likes them but also is willing to work in order to get them.

### History from the Parents

An important part of the psychologist's assessment is an account, from the parents usually but in some cases from a nurse or other caretaker who knows the individual well, of what he is able to do outside the test situation. Besides filling in the background with information that may take time to acquire otherwise —how does he behave in shops? with his brothers and sisters? when frustrated? if he finds a task difficult? if he is scolded? if he is praised? — this account may be especially important in those cases where the psychologist is uncertain as to whether during testing the individual genuinely could not perform an item or whether he was simply unwilling to do so in front of a stranger. Parents are usually thought of as being, if anything, generous in their estimation of their child's abilities but in the writer's experience they are anxious to give as accurate a picture as possible of what he can actually do. What parents say should be taken very seriously, and if this conflicts with what has been observed it is an indication that further observations and tests are required to establish whether or not this particular behaviour really is part of the individual's useful repertoire.

### Experimental Methods

If conventional assessment is rather unfashionable, the use of experimental methods has received powerful support (Mittler, 1973) and the mini-learning experiment has been shown to be of particular value in the assessment of adult mentally handicapped people, whose true abilities may be assessed grossly inaccurately by the usual one-off type of test (Clarke and Clarke, 1973). With children too the best way to determine whether a child is capable of learning a particular skill (given that this is one that is credibly possible for him — no one would attempt to teach a bed-fast child to walk but they might try to teach him to sit up) is to set up an experiment to teach it to him. For example, if a child uses only nouns in speech a programme could be set up to teach him to use verbs. Such an experiment is likely to develop further to the study of what are the optimal conditions under which the child can learn the skill — if he fails under one set of conditions others will be tried — and this too will add to the value of the assessment.

Here the line between assessment and teaching is so finely drawn as to disappear altogether, to the benefit perhaps of both.

**Assessment Procedures: Children**

Although testing is usually carried out in the clinic, hospital or school, many psychologists prefer where possible not to risk a child being upset by unfamiliar surroundings and to test him in his own home. If, however, a multidisciplinary assessment is seen as necessary the child may have to be brought to the centre for testing. Whatever the location the psychologist must decide whether to test the child on his own or in the presence of his parents, or at least that of his mother. Many mothers are eager to see how the child acquits himself while others may be deeply suspicious of the whole assessment process (Shakespeare, 1970) in which case it is preferable for them to see exactly what goes on during testing. A very young child or one who cannot support himself upright in a chair is anyway better tested sitting on his mother's knee, while she will be asked to accompany any child who shows signs of upset at the suggestion that he leave her. The psychologist may ask her to be ready to interpret the child's responses, if these are clear to her and not to the tester, but not to help or prompt him, and most mothers are very co-operative over this. If the mother does not need to accompany the child into the test room she may be glad nevertheless to observe the test session. A one-way screen makes it possible for her to see and hear what is going on without the child being distracted by her presence, while it can be helpful if another member of staff watches the session with her, explains what is going on and discusses with her the purpose of the various procedures.

As with all children, the psychologist will spend some time before embarking on the test in getting to know the child; and will try to ensure that the test conditions are good — that the room is quiet, well-lit, warm and airy, and that the child is comfortably seated at a table that is the right height for him. It may be especially important with a mentally handicapped child to see that the room does not contain too many distractions — flowers, ornaments, pictures — while if he is hyperactive or destructive it may be necessary to remove spare chairs and loop curtains up out of reach before beginning the testing.

During the test itself the psychologist is, to a much greater extent than with a normal child, dependent for the child's co-operation on his enjoyment of the tasks he is doing, and can rely much less on his wish to succeed or to please the examiner. The psychologist then must be especially familiar with the test process, and have all the test materials well organized; one item must follow smoothly on the last, for the child may not tolerate interruptions or delays as the psychologist fumbles for the next piece of test apparatus or hunts for the appropriate place in the recording sheet. Even with a smooth presentation the child may not be able to concentrate for the duration of the full test, and in many cases the testing is spread over two or more sessions.

Since with a mentally handicapped child it is difficult to ensure that he is adequately motivated to do the test the question arises as to how far it is permissible to use extrinsic reinforcers to maintain the child's interest in the tasks. Extrinsic reinforcers have not been used in the standardization of most of the assessment instruments described and consequently their use in testing invalidates the standard procedure (though they could hardly be objected to in the case of the Piaget Sensori-Motor Scales which have not been formally standardized, and are part of the normal procedure with the BAB). Nevertheless the use of incentives may enable a child to demonstrate more fully what he is capable of. Research has shown that when incentives were used during testing they had the effect of increasing the scores only of the more backward children (Clingman and Fowler, 1976) supporting the suggestion that these children are not influenced by the incentives which function for the brighter children, and hence may be unduly disadvantaged by the standard testing procedure.

Many psychologists, faced with the dilemma of, on the one hand, violating the standardization procedure and on the other of possibly underestimating the child's abilities, will give the test first in its standard form and then try the effect of incentives on the child's performance on those items that he failed. The psychologist can then report the child's performance under both standard and varied conditions, and can draw conclusions not only about his abilities but also about his response to the incentives used.

**Assessment Procedures: Adults**

Much of the preceding discussion concerned with children applies also to adults but there are differences of emphasis. Although with adult mentally handicapped people some standardized tests may be used these are seen as less important than the functional and behavioural assessment of skills and deficits, especially in the area of daily living skills. If a person is found to be not fully independent in an area he will be observed over a number of sessions in which he attempts to carry out the task. How much he can and cannot do and any special difficulties will be recorded, and any aspect of the task, where there are environmental difficulties which could be removed, identified (i.e. too tight clothing in a dressing programme). Following this a programme will be set up to teach the skill to him (Moore and Carr, 1976). The result of this kind of approach to the closely related concerns of assessment and treatment is that a developmental model may not be helpful and indeed may need to be ignored. For example, if it would be to a person's benefit to be able to use a telephone, but he cannot read or manage numbers, he would be taught to use a telephone or at least to make the calls he is most likely to need, by the use of any suitable devices — pictures, colour cues, special discs for the telephone dial, etc. — without his having first to master reading and number (Leff, 1974). Appropriate sexual behaviour is also important for the adult mentally handicapped person (Craft and Craft, 1980) especially for those living in the community, and this may need to be taught, from the places and times in which masturbation is acceptable, to social interaction and the skills needed for courtship and marriage (though the latter are more likely to be relevant to the mildly than to the severely mentally handicapped).

### Reports

When the assessment is complete and all the necessary information has been collected, both from parents or caretakers and from others in the multidisciplinary team who have also been concerned in the assessment, the psychologist writes his report. This details the procedures used and any others that may have been given in the past, and the results gained from them, usually in the form of either mental age or quotients; describes the person's behaviour, particularly with a view to deciding whether he appeared to concentrate and co-operate sufficiently well for the test to be considered as giving a valid estimate of his current level of functioning; draws conclusions from the combination of all the data; and sets out recommendations for future action. This report is then circulated to all those involved.

## TREATMENT

The treatment methods to be discussed here are behavioural, as these have had the major impact in the treatment of the mentally handicapped; other methods, such as psychotherapy have sometimes been used with the mildly handicapped (Gunzberg, 1974) — though even with this population their usefulness has been questioned — but are seen as having little relevance for the severely handicapped. Where behavioural approaches are concerned the clinical psychologist has a major role to play in the treatment and management of the mentally handicapped, and will usually be responsible for drawing up and for monitoring programmes, both for individuals and for groups. (Others may of course have this responsibility on occasions or in particular settings — teachers may draw up programmes in their classrooms or specially trained nurses in their own wards.)

### Drawing up a Treatment Programme

Although occasionally the psychologist may expect to take sole charge of the treatment, more often he will be only one amongst many therapists, or may function only as the supervisor of those who will be carrying out the treatment programme. In the latter case he tries to ensure that those who will actually be carrying out the treatment programme — parents or teachers, hospital, hostel or training centre staff, etc — are closely concerned with drawing it up.

The devising of a treatment programme begins with assessment, as already described, to define the problem or problems and to identify possible reinforcers and goes on to specify how, and, perhaps, when and by whom the treatment should be carried out. The problems to be tackled fall into two groups; acceleration targets — those skills that the person lacks and needs to acquire (language, occupation and play, social interaction, self-help skills such as feeding, washing, dressing, and toileting); and deceleration targets — those behaviours that need to be decreased or, hopefully, eliminated (aggression, destructiveness, disruptive, self-injurious and stereotyped behaviours). Although the popular image of the mentally handicapped child stresses behaviour difficulties, in practice the two types of problem have been found, in programmes run by parents, to be quite evenly balanced (Callias and Carr, 1975).

Following on the definition of the target behaviours and the reinforcers the next step in the treatment programme is to define the baseline measures of the frequency or intensity of the target behaviours to be taken before treatment begins, so that these may be compared with similar measures taken during and after treatment. Once these baselines have been taken a second programme is drawn up detailing the treatment methods to be used. For an acceleration target it will specify what will be taught, how often, by whom, what records will be kept, and what are the criteria for success. For a deceleration target the programme will detail what method is to be used when the behaviour occurs, and, if this is a punishment method, how long it will last (for example, if a child is to be timed-out from attention, for how long the adult will turn away from him). Again the therapists will be asked to keep records of when the behaviour occurs and how often the method chosen is used. With either type of programme the psychologist may devise recording sheets tailor-made for a particular programme, although standard record sheets can be applicable in some cases (for example for toileting programmes) while multi-purpose record sheets may be constructed which can be adapted for various purposes.

Where the psychologist himself plans to carry out the treatment it is comparatively simple for him to determine what and how much he will do. When, however, a large part of all of the treatment is to be carried out by others, the psychologist must make sure that the treatment method is acceptable to those who will carry it out; and, as far as possible, that it is feasible to ask them to do so. Much can be achieved by drawing up the treatment programme with the co-operation of those concerned with its implementation, but it is difficult to predict exactly how the treatment will go. It may be necessary to stress that the treatment will be set up on experimental basis and will be reviewed in, say, a week's time or sooner if it runs into difficulties. Staff or parents may be willing to try out a treatment on a limited experimental basis which they would not be willing at the outset to commit themselves to in the long term.

Particular problems may arise where a programme involves the use of tokens, and especially if these are to be used for a group rather than for an individual. Careful planning is essential to determine which behaviours merit a token; the range of back-up reinforcers, how these should be displayed and the exchange rate of tokens for them; the recording method for token delivery and exchange; when and how often the exchange should take place; especially with the more intangible reinforcers such as treats or privileges, how these can be made available and built into the programme. All this may require not only an unusual degree of ingenuity on the part of the psychologist but also that he liaise particularly closely with those who will be carrying out the programme.

In those cases where much or all of the programme is to be implemented by others the psychologist must ensure that they are clear as to what they are going to do, so that as far as possible the programme is carried out consistently. He may need to model the treatment procedure, perhaps in role-play, and then ask the therapists involved to do the same. Once the programme is under way the psychologist monitors its progress; collecting and analysing the records and where appropriate transferring the data on to a graph so that those doing the work can see clearly how it is going. If the programme seems to be working well the psychologist needs only to point this out, congratulate all concerned and leave them to carry on until his next visit. If, however, there has been little progress, or the therapists are unhappy with the programme, the psychologist must reassess it. He looks first to see whether it is really being carried out as specified or whether important errors have crept in which lessen its chances of success. For example, an extinction programme was set up for a child's head-banging but it was found that one therapist, instead of ignoring him when he banged, turned to him and said, 'We're not going to take any notice of that, are we'. If the programme is being carried out appropriately but is still failing to work the psychologist must, in collaboration with the therapists, either adjust the programme or draw up a new one. Long-stay, very difficult people, for whom programme after programme is devised without success, present great problems. The psychologist may feel his head empty of fresh ideas, and yet the person still must be cared for and his problems tackled. Those looking after him can become disheartened and, in the absence of progress, may see the treatment as inappropriate. These objections must be taken very seriously and fully discussed with those concerned, with the aim of reaching agreement on how the person should be handled. Occasionally, where one worker is unable to accept a policy agreed by the rest, it may be necessary for this worker to be absolved temporarily of responsibility for the programme in the interest of consistency of treatment. Where this happens the psychologist must be prepared to deal with feelings of guilt on the part of the resigning worker and of resentment on the part of the others, who may see the worker as having opted out of dealing with a particularly difficult case.

When (as sometimes happens) a programme is working fairly smoothly the psychologist may be able to space out the times he checks on and reviews it, to, say, once a week or once a fortnight especially if the therapists know they can reach him if any emergency arises. At the start of a programme, however, it may be preferable to him to call in after even the first day or two, so that any unexpected difficulties can be sorted out before they become fixed and discouragement sets in.

In this section the treatment discussed has been that of individuals or groups in whom problems, either of learning or of behaviour, have been identified. Psychologists are also much concerned with working for the provision of optimal living and care conditions for handicapped people, which in themselves may help to prevent problems arising. In some instances different systems of care have been instituted (i.e. Kushlick and Cox, 1968) and the effects of these carefully monitored, to enable rationally-based decisions to be taken on the most beneficial system available. Especially for those psychologists working in large institutions, this kind of involvement may be seen as more fruitful use of their time than the kind of crisis intervention described above.

## TEACHING

An important part of the job of a clinical psychologist working in mental handicap is teaching others — other psychologists, nurses, teachers, doctors, social workers, occupational and speech therapists, care staff, and of course parents, and others who may be concerned with a mentally handicapped person. Although the outlook is indeed changing (Clarke and Clarke, 1974) mental handicap has been and to some extent still is an unpopular speciality, so when he is speaking to other professionals the psychologist tries to convey not only information on the history of mental handicap, epidemiology, prevalence, aetiology, treatment and management, but also the idea that mental handicap is an exciting and rewarding field in which to work. His/her responsibilities are perhaps greatest where other psychologists are concerned, as, although there is no lack of applicants for posts in work with normal and disturbed children and adults, posts in mental handicap attract few applicants and may go unfilled for long periods. The situation is improving, however, especially as the psychologist has come to be less of a diagnostician and mental tester. The psychologist-teacher can point to his/her new and more interesting role in treatment and management and to the satisfaction to be gained in seeing change and progress in his or her clients as a consequence of psychological methods of treatment.

Teaching may be by any of the usual methods — lecture, seminar, tutorial, discussion group, etc. (Bligh, 1972; Beard, 1972) — but the psychologist, especially where he is discussing ways of teaching and training the mentally handicapped, makes particular use of practical teaching methods — modelling and role play. The techniques the psychologist advocates may sound simple enough — 'put your hands over his and guide the spoon to his mouth' — but they are open to misinterpretation, and faulty use of them can make them ineffectual. A few minutes of demonstration is worth much verbal or written description, making clear immediately what should be done. So, having discussed with the trainee what he intends to do, the psychologist works with the mentally handicapped child or adult using the method discussed, while the trainee watches. If the method appears to be effective this enables the trainee to embark on using it with increased confidence. If it does not seem to work in this case the psychologist has the chance to review the programme at an early stage, and saves the less experienced therapist from the discouragement of struggling with an ineffective treatment.

Where it is not possible, or perhaps desirable, to demonstrate the method selected on the handicapped person, video-taped examples of the treatment are a good substitute. Video tape may also be used to play back his own performance to the trainee (Bricker *et al.*, 1972) in the presence perhaps of the psychologist who can point to the trainee's successes and, where he is less successful, indicate what might be done differently.

As well as teaching individuals the psychologist is in demand to run courses in the teaching and care of the mentally handicapped. These may be one, three or five day full-time courses or may be part-time and extending over longer periods. The short courses are often for professionals, and, although many different formats are possible, are often run as workshops, with lectures on theory followed by practical role-play sessions. Two tutors work with eight to ten students; one tutor takes the part of the mentally handicapped individual, and the students are asked to 'teach' him carrying out the techniques discussed in the preceding lecture while the other tutor looks on, praises the appropriate things the student does, suggests alternatives to the inappropriate ones, and draws the other students into discussion on the problems involved (Carr, 1980b). Other courses in which the participants meet weekly or fortnightly over a longer period are more often run for parents (Bidder *et al.*, 1975; Callias, 1980; Cunningham and Jeffree, 1971) but also for teachers and other professionals (Smith, 1977; Williams and Jackson, 1975). These follow much the same format as the intensive courses, in some cases with written hand-outs taking the place of lectures. The main difference, however, in these groups is that between meetings the participants take on projects with the children or adults with whom they are concerned; make observations and take baselines, carry out the programmes, and bring to each meeting the record of what has been done since the last. In the practical sessions of the meetings these records are discussed, any necessary adjustments to the programme are made, and the psychologist takes the records away, to analyse and graph the data. (A brave psychologist suggests the parents do their own graphing, teaching them how to do this if necessary.) At the next meeting the psychologist returns the graphs he has made, which provide a clear and, hopefully, encouraging record of progress.

The clinical psychologist sees it as part of his job to evaluate the effectiveness of his work, and this applies also to the training courses. In the simplest form of evaluation the participants are asked to give their opinion of the course's usefulness, often on a structured rating scale. The response, to judge from the published studies at least, is overwhelmingly positive, especially from parents (Cunningham and Jeffree, 1971) with appreciation not only of the group but also of newly acquired skills and experience (Tavormina *et al.*, 1976). Psychologists should perhaps not read too much into this kind of response, since parents especially may be appreciative not so much of the particular kind of course but of the fact that they have received any help at all (Carr, 1980b). Other psychologists have tried to measure more directly the changes in attitudes or skills resulting from training courses, either by written tests or by assessment of practical skills (Bricker *et al.*, 1972) or both (Carr, 1980b; Gardner *et al.*, 1970; Murphy and McArdle, 1978). Evaluation at this level is clearly much to be desired but, since it requires considerable expenditure of time, manpower and resources, may be difficult for the hard-pressed or single-handed psychologist to achieve.

**Research**

As in other areas the clinical psychologist working in mental handicap expects to undertake research, the topics often arising from his clinical work. Most of the major research in mental handicap has come from those for whom their main commitment was not to clinical work (i.e. Tizard, O'Connor, Mittler, Kiernan, etc.) and this is perhaps not surprising in view of the demands put on the clinical psychologist's time. Important research has, however, come from psychologists in clinical posts (Clarke and Clarke, 1974) and there have been many more modest contributions, of which the following are a few examples: Barton, 1975; Callias and Carr, 1975; Clarke, 1960; Dixon and Smith, 1976; Gunzberg, 1974; Murphy *et al.*, 1977; Stephen and Robertson, 1970; Williams, 1978.

**The Work Setting**

Recently psychologists have occasionally been appointed to posts in mental handicap in the community, but the majority still work in hospitals. One of the attractions for psychologists of working in mental handicap is the freedom that they have to decide what form this work shall take. They are seen to have an important role in management (Bender, 1979), and can be directly involved in decisions on admission, treatment, and other organizational policies, and in the way that these policies are determined. Within the hospital then the psychologist works in many different settings — on the wards, in the school, the occupation department or sheltered workshop, in transitional settings designed to prepare the more able patients for independent living. Increasingly psychologists are also extending their work outside the hospital into the community. Those working with children go into pre-school nurseries, playgroups, and schools, to discuss problems with teachers and care staff, to work with them to devise programmes and then to monitor and to modify these if necessary. Staff at hostels for both children and adults look for help from the psychologist in working on difficult behaviours and on ways of teaching essential skills such as self-feeding, dressing, and toileting. Psychologists working with adults may be closely involved with the Adult Training Centres (Whelan, 1977) advising on work and educational programmes, evaluating their effectiveness, and participating in vocational counselling and sex education programmes. Some psychologists have felt dissatisfied with this kind of advisory role and have been appointed to several posts on the staff of hostels or Training Centres; here they feel that they can use their psychological skills more directly to bring about changes in the working of the facilities concerned and in the attitudes and behaviour of other workers; 'there have been many advantages in not being another professional, and . . . (of) working in the day to day situation' (Gray, 1979).

An important aspect of community work in mental handicap, with both children and adults, is concerned with working with parents. 'The great majority of parents wish to keep their mentally subnormal child at home' (Tizard and Grad, 1961); many need help to enable them to do this successfully and many who want to teach and help their own child want to learn how to do this more effectively. Psychologists work with individual parents in their own homes (Howlin *et al.*, 1973) or may run training groups for parents (Attwood, 1977; Cunningham and Jeffree, 1971). An additional advantage for the parents of such groups is that they see, sometimes for the first time, that they are not the only ones with problems, and can learn and get support from each other. Especially if it is not possible for the psychologist or other professionals to continue indefinitely with the group the aim ideally should be that eventually it would carry on independently, with the parents themselves running it, but in practice this has been difficult to achieve.

Other activities the psychologist may undertake depend partly on his own interests and partly on the situation in which he works. Some, working in large long-stay institutions may be much concerned with policy, staff training, and management. Many are committed to working for the transfer of the mentally handicapped from the large institutions, which are seen as not relevant to the needs of these people, and to the setting up of smaller, more educationally orientated establishments, or of even more individualized arrangements such as adoption or fostering, including that of adults and the severely mentally handicapped. Some see the role of the clinical psychologist as described in this chapter as inappropriate to the needs of the mentally handicapped and advocate a radical reappraisal of the role, with predominant involvement in policy making and pressure groups (Dickens, 1978). Others point out that large institutions are not going to disappear overnight and the clinical psychologist has a responsibility for the people still in them (Cullen, 1978). Certainly there is scope for many different approaches and many changes in the psychologist's role may be expected over the next decades.

## CONCLUSIONS

The psychologist's work in mental handicap is widely varied and immensely demanding of his skills, expertise, ingenuity, and energy. In the past his job was regarded as an unattractive one, and to some extent this remains true, with posts left unfilled for long periods (McHatton, 1980). Many probably still feel that little can be done for severely handicapped people but in fact there have been exciting developments over the last few decades. In the 1950s and 1960s the work of Tizard, O'Connor, the Clarkes, and others showed that the moderately handicapped could learn and work at levels previously thought beyond them; in the sixties and seventies it was demonstrated that the severely handicapped could acquire skills with the help of behavioural approaches and benefit from carefully planned programmes of stimulation. These approaches are of some benefit also to the profoundly handicapped, but particular and, sometimes, intractable problems often arise with this group (Remington *et al.*, 1977). This is the challenge for the psychologists of tomorrow; this is where the next major advance in mental handicap must come.

## REFERENCES


Attwood, T. (1977). The Priory parents' workshop. *Child: Care, Health and Development*, **3**, 81–91.

Barton, E. S. (1975). Behaviour modification in the hospital school for the severely subnormal. In C. C. Kiernan and F. P. Woodford (eds), *Behaviour Modification with the Severely Retarded.* Amsterdam: Elsevier North Holland.

Bayley, N. (1969). *Scales of Infant Development*. New York Psychological Corporation.

Beard, R. (1972). *Teaching and Learning in Higher Education.* 2nd ed. Harmondsworth: Penguin Books.

Bender, M. (1979). Overview. Paper given at Castle Priory College seminar. January 5–7, Wallington, Surrey.

Berger, M., and Yule, W. (1972). Cognitive assessment in young children with language delay. In M. Rutter and J. A. M. Martin (eds), *The Child with Delayed Speech.* Clinics in Developmental Medicine. S.I.M.P.

Bidder, R. T., Bryant, G., and Gray, D. D. (1975). Benefits to Down's syndrome children through training their mothers. *Archives of Diseases in Childhood,* **50**, 383–386.

Bligh, D. A. (1972). *What's the Use of Lectures?* Harmondsworth: Penguin Books.

Bricker, W. A., Morgan, D. G., and Grabowski, J. G. (1972). Development and maintenance of a behaviour modification repertoire of cottage attendants through T.V. feedback. *American Journal of Mental Deficiency,* **77**, 128–136.

Brimer, M. A. and Dunn, L. M. (1962). *Manual for the English Picture Vocabulary Test.* Bristol: Educational Evaluation Enterprises.

Callias, M. M. (1980). Teaching parents, teachers and nurses. In W. Yule and J. Carr (eds), *Behaviour Modification for the Mentally Handicapped*. London: Croom Helm.

Callias, M. M., and Carr, J. (1975). Behaviour modification programmes in a community setting. In C. C. Kiernan and F. P. Woodford (eds), *Behaviour Modification with the Severely Retarded*. Amsterdam: Elsevier North Holland.

Carr, J. (1971). A comparative study of the development of mongol and normal children from 0–4 years. Unpublished Ph.D. thesis, University of London.

Carr, J. (1980a). *Helping your Handicapped Child*. Harmondsworth: Penguin.

Carr, J. (1980b). The organisation of short courses. In W. Yule and J. Carr (eds), *Behaviour Modification for the Mentally Handicapped.* London: Croom Helm.

Clarke, D. F. (1960). Visual feedback in the social learning of the subnormal. *Journal of Mental Subnormality,* **IV**, 30–39.

Clarke, A. D. B., and Clarke, A. M. (1973). Assessment and prediction. In P. Mittler (ed.), *Assessment for Learning in the Mentally Handicapped.* London: Churchill Livingstone.

Clarke, A. M., and Clarke, A. D. B. (1974). *Mental Deficiency: The Changing Outlook,* 3rd ed. London: Methuen.

Clingman, J. and Fowler, R. L. (1976), The effects of primary reward on the IQ performance of grade-school children as a function of initial IQ level. *Journal of Applied Behavior Analysis*, **9**, 19–24.

Craft, A., and Craft, M. (1980). Sexuality and the mentally handicapped. In G. B. Simon (ed.), *Modern Management of Mental Handicap: A Manual of Practice*. BIMH MTP Press Ltd.

Cullen, C. (1978). Clinical psychology and mental handicap. Letter to *Bulletin of The British Psychological Society,* **31**, 302.

Cunningham, C. C. and Jeffree, D. M. (1971). *Working with parents: Developing a workshop for parents of young mentally handicapped children*. N. W. Region: NSMHC.

Dickens, P. (1978). The defective psychologists — clinical psychology and mental handicap. *Bulletin of The British Psychological Society,* **31**, 40–41.

Dixon, J., and Smith, P. S. (1976). The use of a pants alarm in daytime toilet training. *British Journal of Mental Subnormality,* **42**, 20–25.

Doll, E. A. (1953). *A Manual for the Vineland Social Maturity Scale: The Measurement of Social Competence.* Minneapolis: Education Test Bureau.

Gardner, J. M., Brust, D., and Watson, L. S. (1970). A scale to measure skill in applying behavior modification techniques to the mentally retarded. *American Journal of Mental Deficiency,* **74**, 617–622.

Garfield, A. and Shakespeare, R. A. (1964). A psychological and developmental study of mentally retarded children with cerebral palsy. *Developmental Medicine and Child Neurology,* **6**, 485–494.

Gray, B. (1979). The psychologist working with mentally handicapped adults in the community. Paper given at Castle Priory College seminar. January 5–7, Wallington, Surrey.

Griffiths, R. (1954). *The Abilities of Babies.* London: University of London Press.

Gunzberg, H. C. (1963). *Progress Assessment Charts.* London: S.E.F.A. Publications Ltd.

Gunzberg, H. C. (1974). Psychotherapy, In A. M. and A. D. B. Clarke (eds), *Mental Deficiency: the Changing Outlook*, 3rd ed., London: Methuen.

Howlin, P., Marchant, R., Rutter, M., Berger, M., Hersov, L., and Yule, W. (1973). A home-based approach to the treatment of autistic children. *Journal of Autism and Childhood Schizophrenia*, **3**, 308–336.

Hurst, J. G. (1962). The meaning and use of different scores obtained between performance on the Stanford Binet Intelligence Scale and the Vineland Social Maturity Scale. *Journal of Clinical Psychology*, **18**, 153–160.

Johnson, R. C. (1970). Prediction of independent functioning and of problem behavior from measures of IQ and SQ. *American Journal of Mental Deficiency,* **74**, 591.

Kazdin, A. E. (1975). *Behavior Modification in Applied Settings*. Homewood, Illinois: Dorsey Press.

Kiernan, C. C. (1974). Behaviour modification. In A. M. Clarke and A. D. B. Clarke (eds.), *Mental Deficiency: the Changing Outlook*, 3rd ed., London: Methuen.

Kiernan, C. C. and Jones, M. (1977). *Behaviour Assessment Battery*. Windsor: NFER.

Kushlick, A., and Cox, G. (1968). Planning services for the subnormal in Wessex. In

J. K. Wing and B. R. Bransby (eds.), *Psychiatric Case Registers*. DHSS Statistical Report Series, No 8. London: HMSO.

Leff, R. B. (1974). Teaching the TMR to dial the telephone. *Mental Retardation,* **12**, (2), 12–13.

Lyle, J. G. (1960). The effect of an institution environment upon the verbal development of imbecile children. III The Brooklands residential family unit. *Journal of Mental Deficiency Research,* **4**, 14–23.

McHatton, M. (1980). Clinical psychologists in mental handicap. *Bulletin of The British Psychological Society,* **33**, 126–127.

Mittler, P. J. (1973). Purposes and principles of assessment. In P. J. Mittler (ed.), *Assessment for Learning in the Mentally Handicapped.* IRMMH Study Group No. 5, Churchill Livingstone.

Moore, P., and Carr, J. (1976). Behaviour modification programme to teach dressing to a severely retarded adolescent. *Nursing Times*, September 2nd, and *Communication*, **11**, (2), 20–27.

Murphy, G. M. (1982). Sensory reinforcement in the mentally retarded and autistic child: A review. *Journal of Autism and Developmental Disorders.* (in press).

Murphy, G. M., and McArdle, M. (1978). Behaviour modification with the retarded: A six month training course for nurses. *Nursing Mirror,* 27th April, 31–34.

Murphy, G. M., and Goodall, E. (1980). Measurement error in direct observations: A comparison of common recording methods. *Behaviour Research and Therapy,* **18**, 147–150.

Murphy, G., Steele, K., Gilligan, T., Yeow, J., and Spare, D. (1977). Teaching a picture language to a non-speaking retarded boy. *Behaviour Research and Therapy*, **15**, 198–201.

Reid, J. B. (1970). Reliability assessment of observation data: A possible methodological problem. *Child Development,* **41**, 1143–1150.

Remington, R. F., Foxen, T. and Hogg, J. (1977). Auditory reinforcement in profoundly retarded multiply handicapped children. *American Journal of Mental Deficiency,* **16**, 279–281.

Shakespeare, R. (1970). Severely subnormal children. In P. Mittler (ed.), *The Psychological Assessment of Mental and Physical Handicaps*. London: Methuen.

Sheridan, M. (1968). *The developmental progress of infants and young children.* (Reports on Public Health and Medical Subjects no. 102), London: HMSO.

Smith, J. (1977). An evaluation of behavioural skills training. Unpublished M. Phil. thesis. Institute of Psychiatry, University of London.

Stephen, E., and Robertson, J. (1970). Paper No. 2. In E. Stephen (ed.), *Residential Care for the Mentally Retarded.*

Stutsman, R. (1931). *Merrill Palmer Scale of Mental Tests.* New York: Harcourt, Brace and World.

Tavormina, J. B., Hampson, R. B., and Luscomb, R. L. (1976). Participant evaluations of the effectiveness of their parent counselling groups. *Mental Retardation*, **14**, (6), 8–9.

Tizard, J. (1960). The residential care of mentally handicapped children. In B. W. Richards (ed.), *Proceedings of the London Conference for the Scientific Study of Mental Deficiency*. Dagenham: May and Baker.

Tizard, J., and Grad, J. C. (1961). *The Mentally Handicapped and their Families: A Social Survey*. London: Oxford University Press.

Wahler, R. G. and Leske, G. (1973). Accurate and inaccurate observer summary reports: Reinforcement theory interpretation and investigation. *Journal of Nervous and Mental Diseases,* **156**, 386–394.

Whelan, E. (1977). Basic work-skills training and vocational counselling of the mentally handicapped. In P. Mittler (ed.), *Research to Practice in Mental Retardation: Vol. II Education and Training.* Baltimore: University Park Press.

Williams, C. (1978). Strategies of intervention with the profoundly retarded visually handicapped child: A brief report of a study of a stereotype. British Psychological Society: Division of Educational and Child Psychology. Occasional Papers 2, No. 2, 68–72.

Williams, C. (1980). The behavioural approach. In G. B. Simon (ed.), *Modern Management of Mental Handicap: A Manual of Practice.* Lancaster: MTP Press.

Williams, C., and Jackson, M. W. (1975). Nurse training in behaviour modification. In C. C. Kiernan and F. P. Woodford (eds), *Behaviour Modification with the Severely Retarded*. Amsterdam: Elsevier North Holland.

Woodward, M. (1959). The behaviour of idiots interpreted by Piaget's theory of sensori-motor development. *British Journal of Educational Psychology,* **29**, 60–71.

Yule, W. (1980). Identifying problems — functional analysis and observational recording techniques. In W. Yule and J. Carr (eds), *Behaviour Modification for the Mentally Handicapped.* London: Croom Helm.

The Practice of Clinical Psychology in Great Britain
Edited by A. Liddell


*Chapter 8*

# *Neuropsychology*

*Edgar Miller*

In its widest sense neuropsychology is much more than a branch of clinical psychology. Neurologists, linguists, speech pathologists, and many others also have a legitimate interest in, and make considerable contributions to, the study of brain–behaviour relationships. This is well illustrated by the fact that a good proportion of the significant texts on neuropsychology that have appeared in recent years have been written by people whose primary disciplinary affiliation is not to psychology.

This chapter is not concerned with neuropsychology as a discipline or sub-discipline. Those wishing to have a general introduction to neuropsychology as a field of study are advised to consult one or more of the recent major texts (for example, Dimond, 1980; Hecaen and Albert, 1978; Heilmann and Valenstein, 1979; Walsh, 1978). In this chapter the focus is upon clinical neuropsychology as it is practised by clinical psychologists who work with neurologically damaged patients. The following sections will first give an extremely brief historical account of the involvement of psychologists in the neurological field in Britain and then go on to discuss in greater detail the work that they do. It will be argued that the emphasis of clinical work in neuropsychology is slowly changing towards a greater involvement in the management and rehabilitation of neurologically impaired patients and that this is the aspect in which clinical psychologists can probably make their most useful practical contribution.

Before passing on to issues of primary concern for this chapter a few further introductory comments may be useful. In general terms neuropsychology is basically concerned with two sets of variables. On the one hand, these relate to the state of the brain after it has suffered some insult due to disease, injury, or surgery and, on the other, to the associated changes in psychological functioning. It can be argued (e.g. Miller, 1972) that the approach to the relationship between these two sets of variables can have either a functional or an anatomical bias. It is possible to examine disturbances produced by disease or damage of the brain in a particular psychological function such as memory or language to see how these might best be described or characterized in psychological terms. This approach can have a more general theoretical interest as well as being important in its own right as a way of better understanding symptoms like amnesia or aphasia. The pattern of breakdown in a function like memory may give insights into how memory processes operate in normal people. In this connection it is interesting that attempts by experimental psychologists to defend the distinction between primary and secondary memory have often appealed to data from amnesic subjects (e.g. Baddeley, 1976). From a practical point of view the better understanding of the functional disturbances involved in neuropsychological impairments could lead to better techniques for ameliorating their impact on the patient's everyday life.

The emphasis of the other approach to neuropsychology is more anatomical. The initial focus is upon a particular structure within the brain. The question then asked is, given a lesion in the frontal lobes, temporal lobes, basal ganglia, etc., what sort of psychological changes are likely to occur? This approach is much more likely to give information which indicates the parts of the brain responsible for different aspects of behaviour. The practical implications of this knowledge are that it may enable features or patterns of behaviour to be used in the diagnosis of the presence and location of brain pathology. It may also be of some interest in rehabilitation since, if the location and extent of a lesion is known, it may then be possible to anticipate the kind of behavioural problems that the patient is likely to encounter.

In Britain there has been a much stronger tendency than in many other countries for the practical or applied aspects of neuropsychology to be concentrated in the hands of clinical psychologists. This does not mean that members of other cognate disciplines have totally ignored neuropsychology. For example, the distinguished neurologist McDonald Critchley often carried out forms of assessment which in many centres would normally be considered the province of the clinical psychologist. Although clinical psychologists are the main practitioners as far as the applications of neuropsychology are concerned it is also true that psychologists working in this field tend to have strong theoretical interests as well. In fact, it is probably the case that, as a general rule, clinical psychologists with a primary interest in neuropsychology are more aware of the academic aspects of their work, and see these as being more directly relevant to clinical practice, than are those working in most other areas of clinical psychology.

## HISTORY

The emergence of clinical psychology as a distinct profession in Britain can probably be traced to the time of the founding of the National Health Service in the late 1940s (although the exact date that is offered will depend upon the definition chosen for a 'distinct profession'). Nevertheless a number of psychologists did carry out significant work in military hospitals during the Second World War. The same general historical picture that is found in clinical psychology in general is also true of that part of the profession concerned with neuropsychology. During the Second World War a few psychologists, such as

R. C. Oldfield and O. L. Zangwill, were fulfilling a neuropsychological role (the latter in the Head Injuries Unit in Edinburgh).

Following the war and with the formation of the NHS psychologists continued to work in neurological and neurosurgical units in civilian hospitals. Among the earliest of these departments was that at the National Hospital for Nervous Diseases in London. Within clinical psychology in Britain neuropsychology has always remained a small specialism and the numbers working predominantly in this field are very much less than those employed in the more traditional areas of adult psychiatry, mental handicap, and work with children. Whilst there can now be very few, if any, psychiatric hospitals that do not at least have a rudimentary clinical psychology service there are still a number of neurological and neurosurgical units without an effective psychological input. Nevertheless the number of these is decreasing and it is fair to say that the slow development of clinical psychology in neurological units has been as much the consequence of the lack of psychologists with the specialized interests and skills as it has been to the refusal of neurologists and neurosurgeons to recognize their value.

## NEUROPSYCHOLOGICAL ASSESSMENT

As with other areas of clinical psychology the original role of the neuropsychologist was conceived as being that of assessment. Unlike other fields neuropsychology is still typically very much orientated towards assessment. In discussing the significance and value of neuropsychological assessment it is useful to distinguish the various goals to which assessment might be directed. In broad terms there appear to be three of these (Miller, 1980a). These are diagnosis, the measurement of change, and the making of decisions about management.

Looking at the literature of clinical psychology of about a quarter of a century ago there was still a considerable interest in tests of 'brain damage'. A prominent example in Britain was Walton and Black's (1957) new word learning test. These tests (see also reviews by Yates, 1954; 1956) were thought to be capable of detecting any 'brain damaged' patient. The assumption implicit in such tests is that 'brain damaged' patients fall into a single coherent group with common psychological features. This assumption has fortunately gradually lost ground amongst clinical psychologists in general but, for the neuropsychologist, it is naîve in the extreme. In fact, the unitary concept of 'brain damage' was largely the product of psychologists working in psychiatric settings. One reason why the unitary concept gained currency and took so long to die may be the very narrow range of brain damaged patients generally encountered in psychiatric settings. Cases of dementia and other forms of generalized cerebral pathology predominate. It is often necessary to discriminate patients with dementia from those with functional psychiatric disorders. In developing tests for this purpose it is easy to slip into regarding these as tests of 'brain damage' in general in the absence of examples of a wider range of neuropsychological impairment.

Disease or injury of the brain can produce a very extensive range of psychological impairments and those exhibited will vary considerably with such factors as whether the pathology is generalized or localized, and if localized, the particular part of the brain that is most affected. The association between aphasia and left hemisphere lesions is one obvious example of this. The kind of pathology can also influence the behavioural picture as can a number of patient characteristics, especially age and handedness (Miller, 1972; Lezak, 1976).

Since the location of any lesion is a very powerful factor in determining the nature of consequent psychological impairments it is reasonable to expect that psychological assessments might be able to give at least some indication as to where pathology might be located in the individual patient. This represents a far more sophisticated means of using neuropsychological assessment in diagnosis than is exhibited by the old tests of 'brain damage'.

It is far beyond the scope of this chapter to attempt even a summary of the various diagnostic tests and techniques in use. Fortunately a comprehensive account has been provided by Lezak (1976). Here there is room for just a few general comments and illustrations.

An influential school of thought in neuropsychological assessment has been that involved in the use of the Halstead–Reitan Battery (see: Lezak, 1976; Reitan and Davison, 1974). This battery is a modified and extended version of the series of tests used by Halstead (1947) in an attempt to measure 'biological intelligence'. The original Halstead battery contained tests of such things as critical flicker fusion, perception of speech sounds, and a finger oscillation test to which Reitan has added other tests including the Wechsler Adult Intelligence Scale, the Trail Making Test, and even the Minnesota Multiphasic Personality Inventory. The whole battery takes several hours to administer and contains what could undoubtedly be regarded as a rather strange collection of measures.

There is no doubt that an impressive range of research has been carried out with the Halstead–Reitan Battery. It can discriminate between groups with different types and loci of lesions (Reitan, 1964) but as Lezak (1976) points out this is usually not at a high enough level for accurate diagnosis with individual patients. Even if it could locate lesions in individuals with a high level of accuracy a battery of this kind would still have considerable limitations. The time required makes it expensive. No matter how accurate the battery is the neurosurgeon opening a head is always likely to prefer the three-dimensional picture of a lesion like a tumour that radiological techniques like the CT scan can give. In addition many of the tests in the Halstead–Reitan Battery have no wider use outside the diagnostic role. What, for example, does it mean for a patient's later readjustment or rehabilitation to know that he has a mild impairment in finger oscillation or critical flicker fusion?

The general comment made in the previous paragraph about the limitations of diagnosis on the basis of psychological changes in view of the surgeon's natural preference for radiological pictures should not be taken as meaning that there are no contributions that can be made to diagnosis by neuropsychology. Consider the following clinical problem. A man in late middle age with a history of heavy smoking is admitted for investigations because of mild signs and symptoms that might be associated with right hemisphere pathology (for example slightly brisker reflexes on the left side and other 'soft' neurological signs). The CT scan shows no definite abnormality but it is well known that small metastases from primary tumours elsewhere in the body (e.g. in the lungs) do not always show up readily on radiological examination. Assuming then that the picture gained from both the standard neurological examination and the CT is equivocal how might the neuropsychologist contribute to resolving the problem?

The first point is that neuropsychological assessment is not likely to answer the question decisively. However, it may very well tip the balance in deciding whether more extensive and invasive investigative techniques like carotid angiography, which also carry a certain morbidity risk, are justified. One approach for the psychologist would be by using the Halstead–Reitan Battery or some other set battery. This may or may not give results consistent with right hemisphere lesions but it still suffers from the limitations set out above. The alternative, favoured by this writer, would be to set up expectancies or hypotheses about the nature of the patient's psychological functioning were he to have a secondary growth in his right hemisphere.

To deal with the problem in this way requires greater flexibility in that the psychologist is not going through the same set assessment routine with each patient. It also requires a knowledge of the kinds of functional disturbance that are likely to be encountered under different circumstances. As far as the present hypothetical case is concerned, it is known that certain kinds of impairment are much more likely to be encountered in subjects with right hemisphere lesions. To cite but one example, Benton *et al.* (1978) have described a simple test of spatial judgement which takes very little time to administer and which is claimed to be selectively sensitive to right hemisphere lesions. In practice more than one test or procedure would be used and testing would continue until strong positive evidence had been found or until it seemed that further investigations would be unlikely to yield such evidence if it had not already been obtained. Of course, the nature of the impairments to be expected would vary with where in the right hemisphere the lesion might be situated and the neurological signs might be helpful in suggesting where the lesion might be within the hemisphere. Possible tests and procedures that might be used have been described (in order of detail) by Warrington (1970), Strub and Black (1977), and by Lezak (1976) with the latter being by far the most comprehensive.

Assessments may be carried out to answer questions other than those related to diagnosis (Miller, 1980a). Impairments associated with neurological damage tend to be long lasting and, although some recovery may occur, a degree of permanent deficit is common. A large number of questions arise as to patient's long-term management and disposal which relate to the degree and nature of the functional impairments. Can a man with a mild aphasia return to his previous work as a salesman where a reasonably high level of verbal facility is required? If not should he undergo some form of occupational retraining and is this possible in view of his coexisting mild memory impairment?

Answering such questions is difficult but often some useful information can be gleaned. Problems like dysphasia and amnesia present obvious problems for readjustment to everyday life. Examining for the presence of dressing apraxia may not only give evidence to help confirm the presence of a parietal lobe lesion but, if the patient is an elderly person who has suffered a stroke, might argue against placement in a local authority home for the elderly which requires a high level of self-help skills from its residents.

An important difficulty in this kind of work is that little is known about how test performance relates to everyday life. It is not known whether the kind of memory difficulties demonstrated by the commonly used clinical tests of memory are the same as those which cause patients and their relatives to complain. In some aspects of functioning correspondence may be very low. The writer and his colleagues have been impressed with the distractibility shown by patients who have suffered severe head injury. This emerges from direct observation of patients working in the Occupational Therapy Department and from the complaints of the patients themselves, their relatives, and employers. This has led to a series of studies aimed at demonstrating this phenomenon under experimental conditions. If successful such a demonstration could lead to a means of detecting those patients likely to be troubled by this problem as well as an experimental analogue which might enable further investigations to be carried out to delineate the circumstances under which distractability might be maximized or minimized. The latter kind of information might be of value in devising means of overcoming the problem.

A preliminary study failed to demonstrate any excess distractability in severely head injured subjects using a card sorting task involving increasing amounts of irrelevant information (Miller and Cruzat, 1981). A further (as yet unpublished) experiment using the Stroop test has also failed to show that severely head injured patients are particularly susceptible to interference from conflicting information. Further work is under way on this intriguing problem. The lesson for the moment is that, in this instance at least, it has proved very difficult indeed to find any controlled way of demonstrating what in real life situations appears to be a serious problem for many head injured patients. It is reasonable to expect that the correspondence between real life impairments and test performance will not be so difficult to demonstrate for other psychological deficits (especially those of language and memory). Nevertheless the fact that such correspondence has yet to be satisfactorily demonstrated poses limitations on any conclusions that can be drawn.

## MANAGEMENT

Neurological injury and disease can produce a wide range of impairments, both physical and psychological, which can have a profound effect on the lives of those people who suffer them. Unfortunately systematic data have not been collected for many conditions. The information that is available indicates that a substantial proportion of those who suffer severe head injuries or rupture of anterior communicating artery aneurysms, and survive, fail to achieve a level of social and occupational readjustment that is consistent with their premorbid level (Logue *et al.*, 1968; Miller, 1979a). As far as head injury is concerned, there is general agreement that the psychological sequelae (memory loss, personality change, etc.) typically present more of a problem for rehabilitation than hemiplegia, epilepsy, and the other common physical handicaps (Bond, 1975).

The problem of rehabilitating those who have neuropsychological impairments therefore presents a considerable challenge for the clinical psychologist working in the neurological field. As yet this area has not received the attention it deserves but interest is increasing. Again, limitations of space prevent a comprehensive discussion of the issues but a more extensive review is provided by Miller (1980b). In this writer's opinion rehabilitation and management have to concentrate on the amelioration of handicaps. In other words trying to find new ways for the patient to achieve the same goals despite his handicaps rather than by trying to recreate lost capacity in memory, verbal functioning, etc. It must be conceded that this is not a universally held view but the reasons for holding it are set out in greater detail in Miller (1978, 1980b). An alternative point of view is expressed by Buffery (1977).

The general philosophy advocated can possibly best be illustrated by a brief case description. The patient was an Accounts Clerk of around 20 years of age who suffered a severe head injury when involved in an accident with his motor cycle. The writer and a colleague became involved with him after the company medical officer had contacted the hospital because of worries about his work performance. Since the work situation represented his major source of difficulty and the employers were extremely co-operative it was possible to examine his work performance in some detail and to try and devise ways of helping the patient in that context.

A number of problem areas were identified. One of these arose because the patient was concerned with the preparation and follow through of bills sent to customers. A customer who wished to complain about or query a bill would often telephone and be put through to the patient if he dealt with that particular geographical area. Usually the patient would be unable to deal with the query immediately but would make some notes on a pad to enable him to do so later. When the time came to do this the patient would find that he had forgotten the details of the complaint or that he had insufficient information from the customer. The reasons for his poor performance appeared to be a mixture of things such as poor memory, lack of concentration, lowered drive and initiative, and a failure to appreciate how far something had to be followed through to meet the standards set by his supervisors.

Rather than tackle this problem by trying to improve his memory or concentration for which no obvious therapeutic techniques exist it was decided to leave the patient as he was and try to provide external props or cues. As far as customers' telephoned queries and complaints were concerned the patient was provided with a notepad containing a set of headings against which he could write the necessary information. It also involved a simple decision tree relating to the nature of the complaint. The patient was then trained to listen to the customer's initial communication of the problem and then to say something like 'Thank you for calling. Just let me make sure that I have got all the details down so that I can look into the matter. Your name is . . . your address is . . . etc.'. This problem was not dealt with as a single case experiment and so no claims are made about the effectiveness of the intervention. The aim is merely to show the kind of approach that can be used.

The two types of disturbance that have provoked most therapeutic interest in the literature are amnesia and aphasia. In the case of memory disorders much interest has been aroused in the possible use of visual imagery. It is well established that the use of visual imagery can enhance the retention of such material as paired associates in normal subjects and a number of studies have demonstrated a similar beneficial effect on retention of learned laboratory type material in patients with memory impairments (e.g. Jones, 1974; Gianutsos and Gianutsos, 1979; Lewinsohn *et al.*, 1977).

Despite these experimental demonstrations of the potential value of imagery, attempts to apply this technique to assist people with amnesic problems in real life situations (for example remembering people's names) have not yet yielded convincing results (e.g. Glasgow *et al.*, 1977). One difficulty is that people with memory problems do not seem to be very good at spontaneously generating suitable images (Crovitz *et al.*, 1979).

It might be thought that the attempts to use imagery go against the general principle set out above that attempts at intervention will be better directed at amelioration than at restitution. In fact this is not so because the use of imagery does nothing to enhance the subject's actual ability to absorb or store information. What it does is to get the subject to use his existing memory capacity in a more efficient way.

There has been a much longer interest in the treatment of aphasia, largely by speech therapists. There have been very few controlled trials of the treatment of dysphasia. Only one has as yet given positive results (Basso *et al.*, 1979). Even here the control was not perfect since subjects were not assigned to treated and untreated groups at random and whether or not the subjects received speech therapy was determined by their ability to get to the clinic for out-patient treatment. There are reasons to suspect that this may have had a significant contaminating effect (Miller, 1980b). Taken as a whole the evidence of effectiveness of the conventional forms of aphasia therapy, including those based upon operant conditioning (Sarno *et al*., 1970), is far from impressive.

There have been attempts to apply psychological and neuropsychological research findings to the treatment of aphasia which may hold out some promise for some patients. The first of these is 'melodic intonation therapy'. This is based on the finding that, in most subjects, the basic functions involved in music seem to be more represented in the right hemisphere whilst speech is a left hemisphere function. Melodic intonation uses singing to mediate expressive speech and so utilizes rhythm or other features of music to cue output. So far this technique has not been submitted to a properly controlled clinical trial but Sparks *et al*. (1974) report that six out of eight aphasic subjects treated in this way showed a positive response despite the fact that they were well beyond the point at which spontaneous recovery could be expected to occur.

Some aphasic patients are left with very little speech consisting possibly of a few isolated words or noises. This is usually described as 'global aphasia'. There have now been several attempts to teach alternative, non-vocal language systems to such patients. This has to some extent been inspired by the apparently successful attempts to teach non-vocal communication systems to chimpanzees (e.g. Premack, 1971). In one series of studies it proved possible to teach five out of eight extremely aphasic subjects to communicate using a system based upon coloured shapes at a level that was better than they could achieve with normal spoken English. The level generally achieved enabled them to answer simple questions, carry out commands, and describe actions. Two of them managed to get a little beyond this.

Although most of the work relating to therapeutic interventions has concentrated on aphasia and disorders of memory other problems have also been tackled. Saan and Schoonbeek (1973) have described an elegant single case study involving the treatment of an accountant with dyscalculia. A group based in New York has concentrated on problems relating to hemianopia and unilateral neglect (e.g. Weinberg *et al.*, 1979).

At the present time the contribution of the psychologist to the rehabilitation and management of patients with neuropsychological impairments is at a very early stage in Britain. It is similarly underdeveloped on the other side of the Atlantic with the exception of just a few centres which appear to have made some systematic attempts to organize this type of work. It is obviously an area in which clinical psychologists working in the neurological and neurosurgical field will become increasingly involved. So far neuropsychologists are at the stage of identifying problems and trying out tentative attempts at solutions. It would be very misleading to suggest that there are any well worked out therapeutic techniques of proven validity.

## RESEARCH

It has already been suggested that psychologists working in the field of neuropsychology tend to have stronger theoretical and academic interests than those whose primary concern is with other aspects of clinical psychology. In this connection it is interesting that one of the most prominent British contributors to research in neuropsychology, Elizabeth Warrington of the National Hospital for Nervous Diseases in London, is an NHS clinical psychologist rather than the holder of an academic post.

Since this chapter is concerned with clinical practice rather than research no survey of research will be carried out. Like other clinical psychologists, and indeed members of the caring professions in general, neuropsychologists have an obligation to evaluate and refine the techniques that they use and to develop new and more effective techniques. This implies a commitment to some forms of research and especially the maintenance of the kind of critical and questioning attitude towards their work on which good clinical research depends.

In neuropsychology there is a gap between what might be described as theoretically oriented research on the one hand and the applied research on the other. For example, a considerable amount of effort has gone into studies of the amnesic syndrome from a theoretical point of view and also into clinical tests of memory. More recently there has been an interest in possible therapeutic techniques for use with patients who have memory impairments. Taken as a whole the theoretical studies show very little relation to the work on the clinical measurement of memory or the management of memory disorders. Whilst some of the practical work on aphasia is better co-ordinated with theoretical ideas significant gaps also exist.

The plea being entered here is that neuropsychologists should not just try to investigate such things as memory impairments by comparing amnesic subjects with normal controls (or other brain damaged groups) in terms of their performance on particular tasks. In addition they should compare groups of impaired subjects under different conditions of, say, learning and retention in order to establish under just what conditions that handicapped subject will perform relatively well or relatively badly. Research of this type is sadly neglected and is much more likely to lead to clinical applications than the traditional style of research (Miller, 1979b). One of the few descriptions of research that could be fitted into this mould is Warrington and Weiskrantz's demonstration that certain kinds of cues could greatly enhance recall in amnesic subjects. This finding was picked up and turned into a therapeutic technique by Jaffe and Katz (1975) in attempting to get a patient with an alcoholic Korsakoff syndrome to acquire new information.

## COMMENT

This chapter has attempted to give a brief and selective description of clinical neuropsychology as it has been, and largely still is. It has also tried to indicate the directions in which it can and should go. Obviously what is presented is one person's personal analysis and opinions. With work on therapeutic intervention just opening up it is difficult to predict what the clinical neuropsychologist will be doing a decade hence. If the past history of clinical psychology in general is anything to go by then the changes over the next few years may well be dramatic.

To date, however, assessment still remains the bread and butter work of the clinical psychologist working in a neurological setting. Whilst the grandiose hopes of test batteries that would identify brain damage and indicate its location and type are undoubtedly misplaced this does not mean that there are not a number of more specific and less extensive questions whose resolution cannot be assisted by appropriate neuropsychological assessment. It would therefore be unfortunate if the known limitations of available assessment techniques and the long overdue but growing interest in possible methods of intervention were to result in the neuropsychologist neglecting legitimate problems of assessment.

## REFERENCES


Baddeley, A. D. (1976). *The Psychology of Memory.* New York: Harper & Row.

Basso, A., Capitani, E., and Vignolo, L. A. (1979). Influence of rehabilitation on language skills in aphasic patients: A controlled study. *Archives of Neurology*, **36**, 190–196.

Benton, A. L., Varney, N. R., and Hamsher, D. de S. (1978). Visuospatial judgement: A clinical test. *Archives of Neurology*, **35**, 364–367.

Bond, M. R. (1975). Assessment of the psychosocial outcome after severe head injury. In R. Porter and D. W. Fitzsimons (eds), *Outcome of Severe Damage to the Central Nervous System.* Ciba Foundation Symposium No. 34. Amsterdam: Elsevier.

Buffery, A. W. H. (1977). Clinical neuropsychology: A review and preview. In S. Rachman (ed.) *Contributions to Medical Psychology.* Oxford: Pergamon.

Crovitz, H. F., Harvey, M. T., and Horn, R. W. (1979). Problems in the acquisition of imagery mnemonics: Three brain damaged cases. *Cortex*, **15**, 225–234.

Dimond, S. J. (1980). *Neuropsychology.* London: Butterworth.

Gianutsos, R., and Gianutsos, J. (1979). Rehabilitating the verbal recall of brain-injured patients by mnemonic training: An experimental demonstration using single-case methodology. *Journal of Clinical Neuropsychology,* **1**, 117–135.

Glasgow, R. E., Zeiss, R. A., Barrera, M. and Lewinsohn, P. M. (1977). Case studies on remediating memory deficits in brain-damaged individuals. *Journal of Clinical Psychology,* **33**, 1049–1054.

Halstead, W. C. (1947). *Brain and Intelligence.* Chicago: University of Chicago Press.

Hecaen, H., and Albert, L. (1978). *Human Neuropsychology.* New York: Wiley.

Heilmann, K. M. and Valenstein, E. (1979). *Clinical Neuropsychology.* New York: Oxford University Press.

Jaffe, P. G., and Katz, A. N. (1975). Attenuating anterograde amnesia in Korsakoff's psychosis. *Journal of Abnormal Psychology,* **84**, 559–562.

Jones, M.K. (1974). Imagery as a mnemonic aid after left temporal lobectomy: Contrast between material specific and generalized memory disorders. *Neuropsychologia,* **12**, 21–40.

Lewinsohn, P. M., Danaher, B. G., and Kikel, S. (1977). Visual imagery as a mnemonic aid for brain injured persons. *Journal of Consulting and Clinical Psychology,* **45**, 717–723.

Lezak, M. (1976). *Neuropsychological Assessment.* New York: Oxford University Press.

Logue, V., Durward, M., Pratt, R. T. C., Piercy, M., and Nixon, W. L. B. (1968). The quality of survival after rupture of anterior cerebral aneurysm. *British Journal of Psychiatry,* **114**, 137–160.

Miller, E. (1972). *Clinical Neuropsychology.* Harmondsworth: Penguin.

Miller, E. (1978). Is amnesia remediable? In M. M. Gruneberg and R. N. Sykes (eds), *Practical Aspects of Memory*. London: Academic Press.

Miller, E. (1979a) The long-term consequences of head injury: A discussion of the evidence with special reference to the preparation of legal reports. *British Journal of Social and Clinical Psychology,* **18**, 87–98.

Miller, E. (1979b). Memory and ageing. In M. M. Gruneberg and P. E. Morris (eds), *Applied Problems in Memory.* London: Academic Press.

Miller, E. (1980a). Cognitive assessment of the older adult. In J. E. Birren and R. B. Sloane (eds), *Handbook of Mental Health and Aging*. Englewood Cliffs, N. J.: Prentice-Hall.

Miller, E. (1980b). Psychological intervention in the management and rehabilitation of neuropsychological impairments. *Behaviour Research and Therapy,* **18**, 527–535.

Miller, E. and Cruzat, A. (1981). A note on the effects of irrelevant information on task performance after mild and severe head injury. *British Journal of Clinical Psychology,* **20**, 69–70.

Premack, D. (1971). Language in chimpanzees. *Science,* **172**, 808–822.

Reitan, R. M. (1964). Psychological deficits resulting from cerebral lesions in man. In J. M. Warren and K. Akert (eds), *The Frontal Granular Cortex and Behavior*. New York: McGraw-Hill.

Reitan, R. M. and Davison, L. A. (1974). *Clinical Neuropsychology: Current Status and Applications.* New York: Wiley.

Saan, R. J. and Schoonbeek, H. R. (1973). Problemen bij de behandelig en de evaluatie van een patient met rekenstoornissen. In A. P. Cassee, P. E. Boeke, and J. J. Barendregt (eds), *Klinische Psychologie in Nederland, Deel 2.* Deventer: van Loghum Slaterus.

Sarno, M. T., Silverman, M. and Sands, E. (1970). Speech therapy and language recovery in severe aphasia. *Journal of Speech and Hearing Research,* **13**, 607–623.

Sparks, R., Helm, N. and Albert, M. (1974). Aphasia rehabilitation resulting from melodic intonation therapy. *Cortex,* **10**, 303–313.

Strub, R. L. and Black, F. W. (1977). *The Mental Status Examination in Neurology.* Philadelphia: F. A. Davis.

Walsh, K. W. (1978). *Neuropsychology: A Clinical Approach.* Edinburgh: Churchill Livingstone.

Walton, D. and Black, D. A. (1957). The validity of a psychological test of brain damage. *British Journal of Medical Psychology,* **20**, 270–279.

Warrington, E. K. (1970). Neurological deficits. In P. J. Mittler (ed.) *The Psychological Assessment of Mental and Physical Handicaps.* London: Methuen.

Weinberg, J., Diller, L., Gordon, W. A., Gerstmann, L. J., Lieberman, A., Lakin, P., Hodges, G., and Ezrachi, O. (1979). Visual scanning training effect on reading-related tasks in acquired right brain damage. *Archives of Physical Medicine and Rehabilitation,* **58**, 479–486.

Yates, A. J. (1954). The validity of some psychological tests of brain damage. *Psychological Bulletin,* **51**, 359–379.

Yates, A. J. (1956). The use of vocabulary in the measurement of intellectual deterioration — a review. *Journal of Mental Science,* **102**, 409–440.

*PART III*

# Development of New Services

The Practice of Clinical Psychology in Great Britain
Edited by A. Liddell


*Chapter 9*

# *Child health*

*William Yule*

It is a moot point whether the practice of clinical psychology in child health settings should be regarded as part of the 'development of specialist groupings'. Indeed, as clinical psychology services develop into the 1980s, the tension between the generic nature of training in clinical psychology and the rapid development of specialist areas of application presents a major challenge to the profession. How this and other tensions to be examined in this chapter are resolved will have a major bearing on the delivery of child health services well into the twenty-first century.

It is the aim of this chapter to examine the need for clinical child psychology services within the National Health Service and to examine how these needs are currently being or might best be met. Inevitably this leads to a critical examination of the training of clinical child psychologists and their career structures. It will be argued that clinical child psychology is an integral part of clinical psychology and, because of its breadth of application, it is not just a 'specialism'. In working towards integrated psychology services for children, it must be recognized that clinical child psychologists differ in orientation and skills from educational psychologists. The existence of two parallel groups of professional psychologists each providing partial psychological services for children cannot be ignored and some of the problems of collaboration will be discussed.

As this chapter is being completed, not only is the NHS facing yet another major reorganization but the British Psychological Society is seeking opinions on the future organization of psychological services for children, both within the NHS and in Local Authority Social Service Departments. Hopefully from these consultations will emerge closer collaboration between different professional groups and different employing authorities. Precisely how any changes will affect services remains unclear. What is relatively clear is the size of the problem facing us and that is a useful place to begin.

## THE IMPLICATIONS OF THE COURT REPORT

Traditionally, child psychology services within the NHS have developed alongside child psychiatry services. As the number of psychologists increased and as their skills became more readily available to medical specialities other than psychiatry, so the range of problems presented to psychologists increased dramatically. It is probably true to say that the bulk of referrals still involve the investigation and treatment of problems, and that psychologists are still not heavily involved in preventive work and health education. Accepting this as a starting point, what sort of problems exist in a typical community and how should psychology services be organized to meet such problems?

Britain has a tradition of undertaking epidemiological studies to help answer such questions. It has long been recognized that waiting lists and other administrative measures give misleading estimates of the need for services. Epidemiological studies of total populations provide much more reliable estimates of the prevalence of different defects, disabilities, and handicaps within a community.

The Court Report (1976) on the Child Health Services summarized the results of a number of reliable surveys, and came to the following conclusions. If one considers the average health district, then it will have approximately 60,000 children under the age of 16 years living within its boundaries. There will be approximately 3,750 children in each yearly age group. Applying the prevalence rates obtained from studies such as the Newcastle-upon-Tyne survey (Miller *et al.*, 1974), the Isle of Wight surveys (Rutter *et al.*, 1970), and the National Child Development Study (Sheridan and Peckham, 1973), the following calculations were made:

> The estimates suggest that about 1,125 children aged 0–4 years will be moderately or severely handicapped by either physical (somatic), motor visual, hearing and communication, or learning disorders which require special health care; 140 of them might need to attend a special school, full-time or part-time according to their age. About 4,125 children of compulsory school age will be similarly handicapped. Of these 700 might need to attend special schools. (paragraph 14.4).

The report emphasizes that these are only approximate numbers and that there will, of course, be considerable variations between districts. Moreover, these figures *do not* include estimates of the numbers of children with behavioural and/or emotional disorders. The report recognizes that minor difficulties are often made worse by adverse social factors, again emphasizing that these figures should only be used as rough guidelines for planning.

Even so, let us consider these figures so far; 5,250 children in the average health district will have some sort of physical handicap and about 850 will need to have some form of special education. This, then, is the level of need in those areas where, in the past, child psychologists have been less active. Of course, not all these children present simultaneously for help. Assuming that problems are identified equally throughout the years, then approximately 225 new pre-school cases will be identified in every year. However, more children with suspected handicap will be seen and this begins to mount up. It could easily mean that 10 new cases should be investigated every week — and what time does that leave for intervention and follow-up?

The Court Committee noted that the

> diagnosis of handicap is not an exclusively medical responsibility, it may require the help of psychological, educational, social work and nursing personnel. The assessment of handicap is a prescription for action — which may be medical, educational or social (paragraph 14.10).

Even so, they recommended that '. . . the primary health care team should provide the main health service contribution in quantitative terms to the diagnosis, assessment and treatment of handicapped children' (paragraph 14.18), and psychologists are not often members of the primary health care team.

The committee recommended that a District Handicap Team be established in each health district and they viewed the setting up of such teams as 'central to our proposals for the comprehensive care of handicapped children' (paragraph 22). Such teams would have both clinical and operational functions. The clinical functions would include the investigation of complex disorders, the provision of advice and support to parents and other professionals within the district, and to liaise with schools. The operational functions were to include the surveying of district needs and the monitoring of services as well as the education of professionals.

> 'The basic staff of this team should comprise a consultant community paediatrician, a nursing officer for handicapped children, a specialist social worker, a principal psychologist and a teacher, together with supporting administrative staff' (paragraph 14.26).

The committee deliberately called for a 'Principal Psychologist' to be a core team member as they wanted to emphasize the importance they show in having a senior and experienced psychologist to provide psychological input. Equally deliberately they did not specify whether that psychologist should be clinical or educational as they felt that they should not get drawn into the disputes between the two professions. The point to note here is that the Court Committee clearly recognized the value of a high level of psychological services for physically handicapped children. What have they to say about psychological services for children with behavioural and emotional problems?

The committee recognized that in discussing psychiatric disorders, they were not dealing with 'illnesses' or 'diseases', but rather with quantitative differences from normality. Emotional disorders and disorder of conduct form the bulk of the problems requiring investigation and treatment, with disorders of development, such as speech delay, enuresis, and learning disorders forming a noticeable proportion of the work load. Epidemiological studies such as those on the Isle of Wight and in Inner London (Rutter *et al.*, 1970; Rutter *et al.*, 1975) indicate that in any one year some 5 to 10 per cent of children have disorders which handicap them in daily life. This level of disorder is considerably greater than can be dealt with by services presently available and organized along traditional child guidance clinic lines.

A partial solution to improving services was seen as an increase in the numbers and an improvement in the training of a variety of professionals, including psychologists.

> Psychologists are particularly needed when emotional or behavioural problems are associated with educational difficulties or developmental delay and when disorders are most likely to benefit from the special treatment techniques developed by psychologists (paragraph 15.15).

One of the reasons for the emphasis on educational difficulties and developmental delay is that children with such problems are known to have a considerably increased risk of also having a behavioural or emotional disorder (Rutter *et al.*, 1970). It is important to bear this overlap in mind. Children are no respectors of inter-professional disputes and in planning services to meet the needs of children, then skills in assessing behaviour and emotion are as essential as are skills in assessing cognition and attainment.

The Court Committee urged that there should be further moves towards integrated child psychology services (paragraph 15.18), but, rightly, did not see it as their function to suggest how this could be achieved. They commented on the training of child psychologists, and this will be returned to later in this chapter. They gave the following advice on the role and location of child psychologists:

> Although their role in inter-disciplinary clinic teams will remain crucial, psychologists also have much to offer in helping children and advising other professionals (such as teachers) outside the clinic setting; we believe that this aspect of their work should be increased. More psychologists should be involved in the assessment and treatment of young children as well as those of school age. It is also necessary that there be a closer liaison between psychological (and indeed all other) services for children and those for school leavers and young adults. The services for older adolescents are particularly weak and need strengthening (paragraph 15.19).

It seems to me that the Court Committee's views on the future of the child Health Services and of the role of child psychology within these services are valuable in guiding any discussion on child psychology services. Not only does the Court Report indicate the extent and the nature of need for services within any community but it also indicates an awareness of some of the problems facing psychology — the division of services between clinical and educational psychologists, the imperfections in training of both groups, the overall lack of trained child psychologists, the need to continue working within multidisciplinary teams while extending independent contributions to other areas. Before examining these problems in turn, what else has DHSS had to say regarding the development and organization of psychology services for children? To discover that, we need to turn to the Trethowan Report on *The Role of Psychologists in the Health Services* (1977).

## IMPLICATIONS OF THE TRETHOWAN REPORT

The Trethowan Committee was established in 1972 'To consider the role of psychologists in the health services'. Their report was drafted by 1974, at a time when the NHS was newly reorganized into 218 Health Districts and there were only 585 whole-time equivalent psychologists. This clearly affected the view the Committee took on possible patterns of organization of psychological services.

> For the majority of the health services with which psychology is associated the focus will be in the District and there would be obvious advantage if psychology could fit into this general pattern . . . for the foreseeable future it is on an Area basis that psychology services will need to be organised. (paragraph 5.3.3)

The Trethowan Committee saw that the first priority of any Area department of clinical psychology should be to continue the development of services in the traditional fields of mental illness and mental handicap. Thereafter, in response to representation from many quarters, there shall be expansion into physical handicap, child and adolescent health problems, neurology and neurosurgery, general medicine, geriatrics, community medicine, and general practice. In order to develop these services, it was recommended that each Area department would have a number of Principal Psychologists each with responsibility for the development of psychological services in particular areas. Obviously, this was a long term aim, but senior grade psychologists should be appointed as soon as possible. One possible way of subdividing services was seen as:

1. Physical handicap
2. Mental handicap
3. Child health
4. Neurological science
5. Mental illness
6. Geriatrics
7. Adolescent services
8. Primary health care

It can be inferred from the description given of each of these eight areas that clinical child psychology would be exclusively involved in two of them (child health and adolescent services), make a major contribution to two others (physical handicap and mental handicap), and some contribution to yet two other areas (neurological science and primary health care). In round terms, clinical child psychology could be seen as contributing to about 50 per cent of the work of psychologists in the health services. Hence one reason for being wary of regarding child psychology as a 'specialism'.

Services for children were singled out for special comment by the Trethowan Committee. They recognized that 'the need for psychological help among children and their families far exceeds what could be provided from the resources of the National Health Service' (paragraph 5.13.1). Teachers, social workers and others need access to psychologists for advice and this has usually come previously from educational psychologists. They saw that, following the Summerfield Report (1968) there would be an increase in the number of educational psychologists who would be more readily accessible to schools and to working with pre-school children. They did not think a convincing case has been made out to bring the two professional groups together and establish a new discipline of child psychology. Instead, they exhorted the two groups to collaborate more closely. Thus, an opportunity was lost for examining in greater detail how such collaboration should be encouraged so as to develop better integrated psychological services for children.

Nevertheless, the Trethowan Report makes the role of psychology services for children central to its overall plan for the organization of psychology services within the NHS. By encouraging the development of co-operation with paediatricians in general hospitals and general practitioners at primary care level, the report recognized many of the initiatives made in these areas. Thus, the stage has been set for clinical child psychologists to work with children and their families in a variety of NHS settings in order to meet a wide range of needs. Before returning to a consideration of how clinical child psychology services might be organized, let us now examine what clinical child psychologists can and might do in the modern NHS.

## SOME PSYCHOLOGICAL CONTRIBUTIONS TO CHILD HEALTH

Throughout childhood, there are many points at which good psychological advice can be helpful in alleviating distress and preventing further difficulties. It is no part of my thesis to suggest that all such advice needs to be given directly by qualified psychologists, but it is desirable both that other health service personnel can turn to psychologists for the advice and that the psychologists are properly trained to give it. Thus, a fully developed District Psychological Service should eventually be able to help with all the problems listed below. No one is suggesting that all probationers should receive experience in all areas.

The earliest point of intervention is during pregnancy. Some women can be identified as being at high risk of having a handicapped child. Increasingly sophisticated obstetric techniques involving ultra-sound scanning, amniocentesis, and various blood tests all contribute to screening for handicaps such as Down's syndrome, spina bifida, or anencephaly. Where a disability is detected, the mother can be offered a therapeutic termination. The danger is that mothers may not be sufficiently psychologically prepared to deal with all the conflicts around these issues. The availability of psychological advice should greatly enhance the quality of the service being offered. Wherever a couple have had a handicapped child, there is a need for genetic counselling and advice on appropriate contraception. Psychological input to such clinics is needed.

Parents appear to benefit from good preparation for labour and delivery. Hospitals have run ante-natal classes for years, as has the National Childbirth Trust. In addition to educating prospective parents on what happens during labour, most classes teach some form of relaxation as an aid to delivery. There is evidence to support the view that good preparation during pregnancy is associated with easier deliveries, the use of fewer drugs in labour and with fewer complications (Doering and Entwisle, 1975; Hennenborn and Cogan, 1975; McNeil and Kaij, 1977). More particularly, there are suggestions that systematic desensitization may be even more effective than general psychoprophylaxis methods in shortening labour and lowering the intensity of pain (Kondaš and Ščentrička, 1972). Since the usual alternative is to use pain-killing drugs which both cloud the mother's consciousness and affect the newborn's level of alertness, it is clearly desirable that psychologists get more involved in this important area.

From a variety of sources, professionals have recently shown more interest in preparing couples for parenthood as a means of preventing later difficulties brought about by faulty child management. Hawkins (1972) has argued that all parents should receive systematic training in child management along behavioural lines. Pugh (1980) summarizes a wider variety of initiations already under way in Britain. Even if only broad goals can be agreed at present, there is still a major problem in determining at what stage in the life cycle such preparation should be given. Of course it should not be a once-and-for-all event, and undoubtedly it would help if all school-children (not just early leavers) were given broader introduction to family life and child care. But teaching parenting skills at a point in time remote from their application may not be effective (Yule, 1980). Introduction to more than feeding and nappy-changing at ante-natal classes would be helpful, and more use of informal groups at child welfare clinics would allow advice to be made available at the point problems were being first manifested. Psychologists now have considerable experience in using behavioural techniques, in particular in training parents to manage a wide variety of children's behaviour problems. Whilst the origins of much of this work is in America, recent studies in Britain show the value of such approaches here (Herbert, 1981; Herbert and Iwaniec, 1981; McAuley and McAuley, 1977; Yule, 1975; Sibisi and Yule, 1982). Closer links between psychologists on the one hand and general practitioners, health visitors, and social workers on the other would ensure that advice on parenting becomes more readily available.

To return to the birth, should the baby be recognized as handicapped there is a need for someone to break the news to both parents as soon as possible. This must not be done hurriedly or on a one-off basis. Parents need to be given information about the nature and extent of their child's disability and must be given time to assimilate it. Personnel in the District Handicap Team have a role in educating other professionals in how best to ensure that parents really get the help and support they need at this time.

As envisaged by the Court Committee, the District Handicap Team could also have the responsibility for ensuring that appropriate intervention was arranged as early as practicable. In this context, at least for severely developmentally delayed children, the detailed materials developed in the Portage Project (Shearer and Shearer, 1972) have proven to be extremely valuable (Revill and Blunden, 1979; Clements *et al.*, 1979). The availability of such materials has proven a great boon, but, as psychologists, we must be careful that the needs of individuals are not overlooked simply because such materials are so readily accessible.

The more psychologists are involved in paediatric assessment clinics, general practice, and well baby clinics, the more they will encounter a wide variety of developmental problems which may not be seen so frequently in child guidance clinics or departments of child psychiatry. Particularly in the early pre-school years, young children present their parents with a bewildering array of difficulties in sleeping, eating, and elimination. Delays in speech and language are more likely to be brought to the notice of family doctors, or at least they are currently more likely to be referred on for specialist help. By their very nature, such developmental difficulties disappear over time, but they can cause untold misery in the interim. Hopefully, psychologists will get much more involved in the investigation and treatment of such problems and it will not be too long until the advice 'Just ignore it, it'll go away' or 'He'll grow out of it' will be seen in its proper perspective.

Many children have special educational needs. As noted earlier, the Court Committee recognized that very young children with severe handicaps will be identified by health service personnel and it is important that representatives of the Local Education Authority are involved at an early stage in planning to meet the children's educational needs. Hence the reason for having a teacher as a full member of the District Handicap Team and for involving psychologists. The younger the child at the time his handicap is identified, the broader the sense in which 'education' has to be interpreted. The need to work along with parents and to provide them with support and advice has already been noted.

With regard to education in schools, the Warnock Report (1978) had a great deal to say about meeting children's special educational needs both in ordinary and in special schools. The main thrust of the Warnock Report was to argue that the existing system of categorizing child handicap was insufficiently flexible to meet their special needs. In response to this, the Education Act (1981) will greatly alter the way in which children's special educational needs are assessed and the role of psychologists in this process. At the time of writing, it has not been announced just what this will entail, but hopefully any legislation will give full recognition to the part which clinical psychologists can play.

Since Circular 2/75 was issued by the Department of Education and Science, educational psychologists have played a greater role in ascertaining children's educational needs. In many parts of England and Wales, it has become customary for whichever psychologist is first involved with the child to complete Form SE3, the psychologist's report on the child. This saves time and unnecessary duplication. Normally, it is rightly an educational psychologist or other responsible officer of the Local Education Authority who completes Form SE4, the summary of recommendation to the Education Officer. Hopefully, even though the forms and procedures will alter, this same spirit of co-operation will continue whatever directives emerge from the Department of Education and Science. Obviously a good deal will depend on good relations at local levels, but clear leads can be given by government departments.

Many children have to go into hospitals, often for painful procedures. Repeated hospital admissions are associated with behaviour problems and learning difficulties later on (Douglas, 1975), but the admissions are probably an index of a variety of social disadvantages rather than being directly causally related to the later sequelae (Quinton and Rutter, 1976). In general, adverse effects of separation can probably be reduced by prior experiences of separation from parents under planned and pleasant circumstances. In particular, adverse effects of hospitalization can be mitigated by the proper preparation of both children and adults for planned admissions. Psychologists have already contributed greatly to novel ways of preparing children for hospitalization (Melamed, 1977). Once in hospital, there are many ways in which hospital routines can be set up to accommodate the needs of children (Lansdown, 1980).

In hospital, most children will be under the care of a paediatrician. As Lansdown (1980) shows, many of the conditions which bring children into hospital have associated psychological aspects which psychologists can best deal with. Psychologists can help with diagnosis and investigations as well as continue basic research into the nature of childhood disorders. However, psychologists are probably best able to help nursing staff over the general management of difficult behaviour, irrespective of the particular medical problem. Whether it be in devising a treatment programme to help a child needing transfusion to overcome his needle-phobia or advising a ward sister on the management of separation anxiety, psychologists have a great deal to offer.

And of course psychologists continue to offer advice to parents when their children are in hospital. Where the child is suffering a life-threatening complaint, work with parents is even more essential. How much should a child be told? How best should parents be supported? Is there a place for group support? The more psychologists get involved in wards, the more such psychologically important questions are raised. The whole area of death and bereavement and the sorts of services required to deal with the problems presented is at long last being considered seriously.

Children also leave home when, for one reason or another, their parents cannot adequately care for them. Usually, they are taken into the care of the Local Authority Social Services Departments. In England and Wales, over 50,000 children are received into care each year (the figure for Scotland being 12,000) (CCETSW, 1978). The largest single reason for children being received into care is short-term illness in the family, although nearly 7 per cent are in care for no other reasons than lack of adequate housing. Nearly 50 per cent of children in care are rated by their teachers or houseparents as having significant emotional or behavioural problems (Yule and Raynes, 1972). houseparents need advice on complex problems of child management and social work managers need consultation on wider organizational aspects of child care.

Increasingly, social services departments are realizing the value of good psychological services. Although there remains a need for psychologists to participate in the assessment of juvenile delinquents, it is increasingly recognized that this traditional function, largely carried out by educational psychologists seconded from Local Education Authorities on a sessional basis, is a poor use of scarce psychological services. Particularly with the advent of techniques of assessment and interaction based on social learning theory, social service departments look to psychologists for more active advice on management. (Brown, 1981; Brown and Christie, 1981) As the Trethowan Report (1977) pointed out, social service departments can indeed ask for help from NHS clinical psychologists. 'Section 11 of the National Health Service Reorganization Act 1973 provides for the services of health services profession to be made available to local authorities . . .' (paragraph 5.3.9). Hopefully, more will avail themselves of this as more clinical child psychologists are appointed.

Finally, children will continue throughout childhood to present to a variety of services with those problems of emotion and conduct which have been the mainstay of psychological services for children these past sixty years. I have examined in detail elsewhere (Yule, 1981) the nature and extent of childhood disorders. It is clear that the time is overdue for psychologists to re-examine these problems and recategorize them from a psychological point of view. Meanwhile, psychologists have made large advances in the treatment of 'child psychiatric' disorders, as is attested to by an examination of a number of recent texts (e.g. Lahey and Kazdin, 1977 onwards; Mash and Terdal, 1981; Ross, 1981; Yule, 1977; Herbert, 1981). Clinical child psychologists require training and experience both in dealing with the wide variety of disorders and in working with co-therapists of different disciplines in a variety of settings.

This leads on to a consideration of how best psychologists should be trained to work with children and their families from within a NHS setting in order best to meet the range of problems detailed above.

## THE TRAINING OF A CLINICAL CHILD PSYCHOLOGIST

This problem has concerned my colleagues and me for many years. It has long been recognized that initial two-year postgraduate degree training or three-year in-service training are both insufficient fully to equip clinical psychologists to fulfil all the functions required of a psychologist working with children. But, then, initial training is only an introduction to the profession and basic grade is still essentially a training grade. By careful selection of options and placements, a number of trainees can gain considerable supervised experience with a variety of child clients, whilst at the same time having experience of adult patients within the NHS. The generic aspects of training are highly valued and allow a clinical child psychologist to work with adult patients as well as to understand the neurophysiological basis of many cognitive problems. Moreover, virtually all clinical psychologists are taught in multidisciplinary settings and this is invaluable in participating in multidisciplinary teams later. Even so, the basic disciplines of child psychology have expanded at such a rate that it is difficult to do the subject justice in the confines of present training (Berger, 1975).

Some years ago, Dr Berger and I argued that there was an urgent need to improve the standard of applied child psychology available in the NHS (Berger and Yule, 1975). Regarding child psychologists as applied scientists, we argued that in addition to having a detailed knowledge of child and adolescent psychology and the phenomenology of children's problems, what was required was a good grasp of appropriate research methodology, assessment, treatment, and the understanding of the structure and organization of services. We put forward detailed proposals for the syllabus of a one-year course which could be taken as a post-qualifying course after at least one year on basic grade. We made the 'mistake' of suggesting that such a course would be open to educational and research psychologists, and the repercussions of that suggestion are still reverberating through the British Psychological Society's sub-systems. Despite this, I stand by the basic premise which is that currently neither clinical nor educational psychologists are sufficiently trained by their initial training to provide a comprehensive psychological service for children.

The outline syllabus proposed by Berger and myself is given in the Appendix. I believe that this can still form the basis for post-qualification courses, the need for which is now widely recognized within the profession.

Strategically, however, it is clear from the number of advertisements which appear that there is still a large need for well-qualified basic grade psychologists to work with children. All the courses need to ensure that they are able to provide sufficient and sufficiently varied supervised experience of working with children and adolescents. Whilst some of this should continue to be within a child psychiatry setting, this is not mandatory under current British Psychological Society regulations. Greater advantage should be taken of the increasing opportunities to work in paediatric settings.

Returning to post-qualification training, not only is there an urgent need for a variety of short and long term courses, but there is also a need to examine how funding for such training can best be obtained. The 'medical model' of disease is rightly reviled by many psychologists, but the 'medical model' of continuing education has been largely ignored. Our profession needs to have provisions for paying for short courses, for paying for secondments of up to a year, and for the establishment of post-qualification training places. Until this is fully worked out, we will be unable to develop our skills to the full advantage of the country's children. This need has been recognized by the recent British Psychological Society Working Party on 'Psychological Services for Children' (1981).

## SOME CURRENT AND RECURRING PROBLEMS

Earlier in this chapter I have touched on a number of professional issues which apply particularly to those of us working with children within the NHS. Let me now examine each of them briefly.

### 1 A 'Specialism'

At the outset, I said that I was not too happy with clinical child psychology being regarded as a 'specialism'. That is not to say that psychologists working with children do not require a great deal of special knowledge. The critical thing is the extent to which their core professional skills are shared with other clinical psychologists. Of course, clinical child psychologists are 'marked off' by working with one identified group of clients — who form a very large proportion of the total population. Their needs and problems differ in content from those of adult patients but they are not in any way fewer or more 'specialized'. Thus if 'specialism' is intended to denote 'less general', then I repute the usage.

As I noted earlier, child psychologists have contributions to make to six of the eight areas of practice differentiated in the Trethowan Report. Again, if 'specialism' means 'minority application', child psychologists are not specialists. If 'specialist' means well-trained, fully professional and able to deal with the majority of the problems described in earlier sections, then I will admit of clinical child psychologists having aspirations to being regarded as specialists.

My concern here is not merely a semantic one. Our profession has recently reasserted its belief in the value of the initial generic training shared by clinical psychologists. As I noted, I believe that our exposure to adult patients, to neurophysiology, to other professions in training, all of these contribute to our ability to deal with the varied challenges to be met in the NHS. There is a danger that if child psychology is seen as a specialism, then there may be attempts in some quarters to teach it separately from other aspects of clinical psychology, and I think that would not be in the interests of NHS clients.

I have another worry and that concerns promotional prospects for people who specialize in working with children. The number of Principal posts in this area is growing at a gratifying rate. However, in recent years I have seen too many Area Principal or Top grade posts where the administrative promotion is tied to clinical work with adult patients — thereby effectively blocking psychologists who work with children from promotion. I sometimes get the feeling that 'adult psychologists' are seen as able to supervise 'child psychologists' but not vice versa. In so far as a specialist label contributes to this false perception, it should be avoided.

### 2 Relations with Educational Psychology

From the age of 5 to 16, all children are required to attend school (or receive satisfactory education otherwise). All Local Education Authorities now employ educational psychologists and provide schools psychological services. Despite the amazing growth in the number of educational psychologists throughout the 1970s, there are still too few psychologists — either clinical or educational — working with children.

According to the BPS working party (BPS, 1981) 311 educational psychologists are employed in Scotland and 1037 in England and Wales. Within the NHS, out of a total of 1,100 clinical psychologists, approximately 300 work with children, including handicapped children. About half of these only work part-time with children. Thus, clinical child psychologists are already providing a sizeable amount of service to children. We know from epidemiological studies that if all child psychiatric services were to rely on school referrals by teachers, then 50 per cent of the children requiring help would not be identified (Rutter *et al.*, 1970). Many parents discuss their difficulties with their GPs and access the rest of the NHS that way. Thus, it is obvious that the need for child psychology services within the NHS will continue.

A recent court case involving an educational psychologist in dispute with his employers, has been interpreted by Sutton (1981) as demonstrating that educational psychologists must conform to their employers' instructions. In other words, their degree of professional independence is not as wide as was believed. This has serious implications when one realizes that parents often wish to turn to psychologists for advice on school problems — advice they hope will be independent of local authority policies. Doubtless clinical psychologists are also constrained by their terms of employment, but perhaps it is a blessing in disguise for the families of our clients that they can turn to the other group when they want a second, truly independent opinion.

Be that as it may, it is likely that the two professions will grow in parallel and that services to children will improve. There are clear needs for formal and informal liaison between the psychologists providing services within a district — the exact form of collaboration will depend on local circumstances. The BPS working party's (1981) recommendation that Area Groups of Psychological Services for Children be set up has much merit and hopefully will succeed in promoting even greater co-operation between the disciplines.

## 3 Multidisciplinary Team

Child psychologists are used to working in multidisciplinary teams, largely taking over the role structures from early child guidance days (Sampson, 1980). There is a great deal to be said for bringing together the views of different disciplines when trying to understand the complex problems of children presented from within complex social networks. Most of us who have worked in such a way can appreciate its strengths. But there are also weaknesses.

The different team members all too frequently are accorded different status (and salaries) which bear no relation to their experiences or expertise. Too often the medical member espouses the hollow doctrine of *primum inter pares*.

The system has been vigorously criticized by sociological analysts and equally vigorously attacked on pragmatic grounds (Tizard, 1973). Structural changes in the provision of services have dealt heavy blows against the notion of permanent teams and substituted the concept of shifting networks of services (DES, 1974).

In my view, whilst it is important that the independent professional contribution of clinical child psychologists is properly recognized, it would be foolish to deny the value of interdisciplinary collaboration. Psychologists are, and should remain, accountable through other psychologists to their employers, but that is not to say that they should not work closely with other disciplines. Hopefully we will see the emergence of proper child psychology clinics to which other disciplines provide consultation as requested, in the same way as psychological consultation is currently provided to medical and social work clinics.

The British Psychological Society Working Party on Psychological Services for Children (BPS, 1981) put forward the unusual concept of the need to define Independent Professional Status with respect to psychological work with children. Not surprisingly this has already been disavowed by the Division of Clinical Psychology who prefer to keep the profession generic. All clinical psychologists exercise independent professional judgement once they reach senior grade. The need for the concept was introduced after complex discussion with child psychiatrists and psychiatric social workers on the future of training for work in child guidance clinics. No need to guess which profession attained 'Independent Professional Status' earliest! I suggest, rather than waste precious professional time debating such status issues, psychologists should continue to improve their skills and allow sapiential authority to develop where status may lag behind.

## 4 Organization of Services

Even allowing for an estimated 150 full-time equivalent child psychologists being in posts in about 200 district health authorities, not only are many of these working in mental handicap but many of the others work in and around London. In other words, there are too few people inequably distributed to begin to decide an optional organization for services. Now that services are to be reorganized at District level, the role of Regional Speciality or organizing committees will be increased. It will be essential for clinical child psychologists to co-operate throughout regions on plans to develop adequate services at a time when little growth is to be expected.

Taking this gloomy, but realistic, view, the advice of the Trethowan Report remains valid. Priority has to be given to developing services in child psychology and mental handicap before branching into newer areas. That does not mean that all sessions in an understaffed service have to be committed to those areas, only that relatively speaking it is advisable to give those areas some priority. Simultaneously, any good Senior or Principal will be providing occasional sessions in other services to broaden experience and gain a feel for the likely level of future demand.

It is vital that as many trainees as possible are given excellent child health experience as early as possible so that more can elect to take extra placements with children during preliminary training. That way district services can build up a pool of experienced basic grades on whom future expansion will depend.

## A FINAL WORD

This chapter has concentrated on the organizational and policy aspects of providing psychological services for children. Since it could not have done justice to the vast new literature on applications of child psychology to children's problems it has not attempted even a superficial coverage. It has assumed that clinical psychologists do not need to be convinced of the potential value of improving child psychology services within the NHS. Instead, it has tried to discuss the broad nature of problems presenting within the child health services. It has recognized that there are many organizational problems ahead, not the least being the improvement of collaboration with educational psychology colleagues.

Children *are* different from adults. Working with children is more demanding in many ways. Not only are they developing rapidly, they are also inextricably involved in a variety of social networks. Therein lies one of the challenges for an applied child psychologist. With the burgeoning interest in child development, the nature of the work will change dramatically in the next decade. It is up to all of us to ensure that, built on those developments, the services to our clients really improve.

## ACKNOWLEDGEMENTS

I would like to acknowledge the many hours of discussion with Dr Michael Berger which have greatly influenced my thinking on services for children. I also remain indebted to my tutor and friend, the late Professor Jack Tizard.

## REFERENCES

Berger, M. (1975). Clinical psychology services for children. *Bulletin of The British Psychological Society,* **28**, 102–107.

Berger, M. (1977). Psychology in paediatrics and child care. In S. Rachman (ed.), *Contributions to Medical Psychology: Vol I.* Oxford: Penguin.

Berger, M., and Yule, W. (1975). Proposals for the training of child psychologists. Unpublished paper presented to the Division of Clinical Psychology, British Psychological Society.

British Psychological Society (1981). *Psychological services for children.* Leicester: BPS.

Brown, B. (1981). A constructive role for assessment. *Concern,* **40**, 5–8.

Brown, B., and Christie, M. (1981). *Social Learning Practice.* Oxford: Pergamon.

Central Council for Education and Training in Social Work (1978). *Good Enough*

*Parenting: Report of a group work with children and young people and the implication for Social Work Education.* London: CCETSW.

Clements, J. C., Bidder, R. T., Gardner, S., Bryant, G., and Gray, O. P. (1979). A home advisory service for pre-school children with developmental delays. *Child: Care, Health and Development,* **6**, 25–33.

Court, S. D. M. (1976). *Fit for the Future: Report of the Committee on Child Health Services.* London: HMSO.

Department of Education and Science (1974). Child Guidance — Circular 3/74. London: HMSO.

Department of Education and Science (1975). The discovery of children requiring special education and the assessment of their needs. Circular 2/75. London: HMSO.

Doering, S. G., and Entwisle, D. R. (1975). Preparation during pregnancy and ability to cope with labor and delivery. *American Journal of Orthopsychiatry,* **45**, 825–837.

Douglas, J. W. B. (1975). Early hospital admissions and later disturbances of behaviour and learning. *Developmental Medicine and Child Neurology,* **17**, 456–480.

Hawkins, R. P. (1972). It's time we taught the young how to be good parents (and don't you wish we'd started a long time ago?). *Psychology Today*, pp. 28, 30, 36, 38–40.

Henneborn, W. J., and Cogan, R. (1975). The effect of husband participation in reported pain and the probability of medication during labor and birth. *Journal of Psychosomatic Research,* **19**, 215–222.

Herbert, M. (1981). *Behavioural Treatment of Problem Children: A Practice Manual.* London: Academic Press.

Herbert, M., and Iwaniec, D. (1981). Behavioural psychotherapy in natural home settings: An empirical study applied to conduct disordered and incontinent children. *Behavioural Psychotherapy,* **9**, 55–76.

Kondaš, O., and Ščentrická, B. (1972). Systematic desensitization as a method of preparation for childbirth. *Journal of Behaviour Therapy and Experimental Psychiatry,* **3**, 51–54.

Lahey, B. B., and Kazdin, A. E. (1977 onwards). *Advances in Clinical Child Psychology Vols 1–4*. New York: Plenum.

Lansdown, R. (1980). *More Than Sympathy.* London: Tavistock.

Mash, E. J., and Terdal, L. G. (eds) (1981). *Behavioral Assessment of Childhood Disorders.* New York: Guildford Press.

McAuley, R. and McAuley, P. (1977). *Child Behaviour Problems: An Empirical Approach to Management.* London: Macmillan.

McNeil, T. F., and Kaij, L. (1977). Prenatal, perinatal and post-partum factors in primary prevention of psychopathology of offspring. In G. W. Albee and J. M. Joffe (eds), *Primary Prevention of Psychopathology: Vol I: The Issues*. Hannover, New Hampshire: University New England Press.

Melamed, B. G. (1977). Psychological preparation for hospitalization. In S. Rachman (ed.), *Contributions to Medical Psychology: Vol I.* Oxford: Pergamon.

Miller, F. J. W., Court, S. D. M., Knox, E. G., and Brandon, S. (1974) *The School Years in Newcastle upon Tyne.* London: Oxford University Press.

Pugh, G. (ed.) (1980). *Preparation for Parenthood: Some Current Initiatives and Thinking.* London: National Children's Bureau.

Quinton, D., and Rutter, M. (1976). Early hospital admissions and later disturbances of behaviour: An attempted replication of Douglas' findings. *Developmental Medicine and Child Neurology,* **18**, 447–459.

Revill, S., and Blunden, R. (1979). A home training service for pre-school developmentally handicapped children. *Behaviour Research and Therapy,* **17**, 207–214.

Ross, A. O. (1981). *Child Behavior Therapy.* New York: Wiley.

Rutter, M., Cox, A., Tupling, C., Berger, M., and Yule, W. (1975). Attainment and adjustment in two geographical areas. I: The prevalence of psychiatric disorders. *British Journal of Psychiatry,* **126**, 493–509.

Rutter, M., Tizard, J., and Whitmore, K. (eds.), (1970). *Education Health and Behaviour*. London: Longman.
Sampson, O. (1980). *Child Guidance: Its History, Provenance and Future.* Leicester: BPS.
Shearer, M. S., and Shearer, D. E. (1972). The Portage Project: A model for early childhood education. *Exceptional Children,* **39**, 210–217.
Sheridan, M., and Peckham, C. (1973). Hearing and speech at seven. *Special Education,* **62**, 16–20.
Sibisi, T. Y., and Yule, W. (1982). Parent training in a small group: A pilot study. *Child: Care, Health and Development*, **8**, 141–150.
Summerfield, A. (1968). *Psychologists in Education Services.* London: HMSO.
Sutton, A. (1981). Whose psychology? Some issues in the social control of psychological practice. In I. McPherson and A. Sutton (eds), *Reconstructing Psychological Practice.* London: Croom Helm.
Tizard, J. (1973). Maladjusted children and the child guidance service. *London Education Review,* **2**, 22–37.
Trethowan, W. H. (1977). *The Role of Psychologists in the Health Services.* London: HMSO.
Warnock, M. (1978). *Special Education Needs.* London: HMSO.
Yule, W. (1975). Training parents in child management. *Journal of the Association of Educational Psychologists,* **10**, 11–15.
Yule, W. (1977). Behavioural approaches to treatment. In M. Rutter and L. Hersov (eds), *Child Psychiatry: Modern Approaches.* Oxford: Blackwell.
Yule, W. (1980). Verhaltens modifikationen in Kindesalter: Moglichkeiten der Pravention (Behaviour modification in childhood: Possibilities of prevention). Chapter 6 In P. F. Schlottke and H. Wetzel (eds), *Psychologische Behandlung von Kinden und Jugendlichen.* Munchen: Urban and Schwarzenberg.
Yule, W. (1981). The epidemiology of child psychopathology. In B. B. Lahey and A. E. Kazdin (eds), *Advances in Clinical Psychology Psychology: Vol 4.* New York: Plenum.
Yule, W., and Raynes, N. V. (1972). Behavioural characteristics of children in residential care in relation to indices of separation. *Journal of Child Psychology and Psychiatry,* **13**, 249–258.

# APPENDIX

## The Content of Focused Training

The content outlined below is intended to provide a basis for the development of practical applications of psychological research. Indeed, it is the constant emphasis on such applications which will provide one of the major justifications for focused training.

The following outline indicates specific topics to be covered in a training programme. While it may appear to be over-inclusive candidates will already have covered a substantial proportion of the topics in their previous training. Hence, courses will have to be flexible enough to cope with individual experience, cater for the development of individual interests and needs, yet ensure that they leave the course with a core of common knowledge and practical experience.

*Section A*: Child Development and Adolescent Psychology

1 The Psychology of Development
To include an introduction to:
Genetics, particularly behaviour genetics
Neuroanatomy, neurophysiology, and psychophysiology
Physical growth and change
Neuropsychology
2 Individual Development
To include:
Sensory processes
Motor development
Conditioning and learning
Perception
Cognition
Attention
Motivation and emotion
Personality and individual differences
Speech and language
3 Socialization
Interaction and attachment
Family influences
Peer group
School
Cultural differences and their implications
4 Theories and Models of Child and Adolescent Development
Approaches to the study of child development
Mechanistic and organismic theories
Stage and phase theories
Specific theories — including Piaget, social learning, etc.
5 Integration of Topics covered in Sections 1 to 4

This section is intended as an integration of the material covered above. Its goal is to describe the interrelationships among various mechanisms and processes at different phases of the life-span.

Pre-natal development
Post-natal (neonate and infant)
The first two years
Pre-school
Middle childhood
Adolescence

*Section B1*: Clinical Orientation and Phenomenology

To include:
Paediatrics

Adult, adolescent and child psychiatry
Neurology, including paediatric neurology
Orthopaedics
Ophthalmology
E.N.T.
Dentistry

The purpose of introducing these medical aspects is to alert child psychologists to the major medical conditions which afflict children and adolescents with special reference to their associated psychological difficulties. Some of these topics should be given more weight than others (for example, child and adolescent psychiatry), and some should be complemented by psychological approaches where these are available (for example, neurology complemented by neuropsychology).

Aetiological aspects

- Genetic and constitutional
- Endocrine
- Metabolic
- Infectious
- Traumatic injury
- Malnutrition, neglect, and child abuse
- Familial and social factors
- Temperament

Phenomenology

To include:

- Sensory and motor defects
- Cognitive (intellectual/educational; reading, writing, spelling, number, etc.)
- Emotional
- Social
- Language
- Single and multiple handicap (the overlap and interaction of handicaps)
- Giftedness and special abilities

*Section B2*: Associated Problems

To include:

- Psychopharmacology
- Hospitalization, physical and psychological aspects
- Preparation for surgery and aftercare
- Institutionalization, physical and psychological aspects
- Doctor – patient – parent communication
- Treatment and the problems associated with failure to follow advice/utilize professional help/services
- Health education and propaganda

*Section C*: Statistics and Research Methods

To include:
Methodology
Research design and statistics
Introduction to multivariate analysis and Bayesian statistics
Single case research and 'statistics'
The evaluation of intervention and services
Translating research problems into actual studies, with special emphasis on applied research
The determination of service needs
The use of computers

*Section D*: Assessment Procedures

To include:
Test design, construction and evaluation
Test procedures: (a) conventional — baby tests, intelligence attainments, language, motor functioning.
(b) an extension of the concept of 'test', involving the use of:

direct observation procedures
interviewing
neuropsychological procedures
psychophysiological measurement, biofeedback
conditioning techniques as tests, habituation procedures
techniques for the evaluation of quality of care
the utilization of research techniques as 'tests', for example the measurement of attention, impulsivity, reaction time using techniques and findings of published studies
Testing and assessment and their relationship to treatment

*Section E*: Treatment

Behavioural approaches
Counselling
Psychodynamic approaches
Educational approaches — including remedial techniques
Working with families
Ethical problems in treatment
Parents and other non-psychologists as therapists
Rehabilitation, and the integration of individuals with special needs into the general community
Coping with the transition between various forms of special care

Where possible teaching should include demonstrations in the form of video and audio recordings, role playing and mini-workshops

*Section F*: Legislation, Services, and Institutions

1. Legislation concerning children and regional variations (Scotland, Ireland and Wales), Education, Adoption, Fostering, Care.
2. National organization
   DHSS, DES, Home Office, Structure in Scotland, Ireland and Wales.
3. Regional structure and organization
   NHS Areas, etc.
   DES Structures (e.g. School Health)
   Local Authority (Education, Social Services, Health Structures, Child Minding, Fostering, Playgroups, Nursery Schools etc.)
4. 'Charitable' organizations concerned with children, for example NSPCC, Spastics Society, NAMH, IRMH, Autistic Society, etc.
5. Research units (e.g. MRC), Sponsoring organizations (SSRC)
6. Professions associated with child health and care GP, Midwives, Health Visitors, Nurses, Speech Therapists, Physiotherapists, Occupational Therapists, Child Care Staff, Social Workers, Probation Officers, School Counsellors.
7. The social psychology of management, administration and institutional change.
8. The 'Politics of Services': for example using the Autistic Society as a case study.
9. Co-operation with governmental and other agencies aimed at effecting policy changes.

*Section G*: Practical Experience

The practical work should be planned so as to avoid spectator placements: it is essential to ensure that candidates are actively involved in the on-going work. Given that they already have had some practical experience, candidates will be able to contribute to the on-going work in their placements.

1 Assessment

To include the following, preferably as part of 'clinical' work:

The administration of conventional tests

The administration of other procedures as 'tests', such as GSR, direct observation procedures, quality of care measures.

Development and use of specially designed tests

2. Treatment and intervention: individual, group, and institutional

To include:

The planning and implementation of a variety of treatment regimes, for example behavioural with individual/parent training; counselling with adolescent; 'remedial' reading, maths, etc.

3. Detailed case studies of instances of institutional change, for example Brooklands experiment; Southampton Services.

4 Placements

There should be a minimum of three months in a number of supervised settings, determined in part by the individual's previous experience.

*Essential:*

Paediatric
Social Services

*Optional (Choice of two, depending on initial training/experience)*

Subnormality
Psychiatric
L E A Clinic
Community/Group General Practice

*Section H*: Area of Special Interest

The course should provide the opportunity for individual members to work intensively in an area that is of special interest to them, both at an academic and a practical/research level.

Many of the candidates will have had the opportunity during their initial professional or other courses to complete a small research project. While on the proposed course, they should undertake a research project which has practical implications. It will be necessary to provide certain back-up resources, such as technical help, funding for equipment, etc.

The Practice of Clinical Psychology in Great Britain
Edited by A. Liddell


*Chapter 10*

# *Adolescent services*

*Dorothy M. Fielding*

The Court Report on child health services in the United Kingdom (DHSS, 1976) begins its chapter on adolescents with the following statement 'In recent years it has become increasingly evident that adolescents have needs and problems sufficiently distinguishable from those of adults to warrant consideration as a distinct group for health care provision' (p. 163). The report goes on to describe some of the special needs of adolescents within health service settings. For example, it notes that the facilities available for physically ill adolescents at hospital level are those primarily provided for children or adults. Accordingly, a mature adolescent might find himself or herself on a children's ward where the ward routine is inappropriate. Conversely, an immature fourteen-year-old might be found in the unsuitable environment of an adult ward. The report concludes that improved facilities for adolescents are needed. Moreover, it recommends that particular attention be given to provision for the psychological and emotional problems of adolescence (paragraph 11.11, p. 167). A year later the Trethowan Committee (DHSS, 1977) recommended that one of the specialist divisions within an area department of clinical psychology should be solely responsible for adolescent services and that the head of the section should ideally be of principal psychologist status.

Both of these reports draw attention to the special needs of the adolescent patient. Such attention is welcome since their needs have often been neglected in favour of the development of child or adult services. It is the purpose of this chapter first to outline some of the problems and needs of adolescent youngsters and secondly to describe some of the approaches taken by clinical psychologists working within different health service settings to meet these needs. Finally, the chapter comments upon areas for future development within adolescent clinical psychology services. However, before addressing these issues directly it is necessary to consider what constitutes the adolescent period and to describe how this period may be differentiated from other stages of development.

## THE ADOLESCENT PERIOD — A DEFINITION

Adolescence is often defined as the 'growing up period between childhood and maturity' (Graham and Rutter, 1976). However, this simple definition conceals a number of issues which require more detailed elaboration. In the first place problems arise in the selection of the criteria adopted to delineate the end of childhood or the beginning of adulthood. The major physical changes of puberty are usually taken to indicate the starting point for adolescence. In particular the onset of menstruation in girls and the appearance of pubic hairs in boys are used to signify the beginning of puberty and the end of childhood. However, the choice of these events is to some extent arbitrary since these two easily observable changes form only a small part of the complex bodily modifications taking place around this time.

Similar difficulties arise in defining the upper limit of adolescence. Clearly a number of criteria could be adopted, for example the attainment of physical or emotional maturity or simply arrival of the statutory age at which adult responsibilities can be taken on (e.g. voting, marriage, etc.).

A second problem in the definition of the adolescent period arises from the considerable variability in the age at which individuals achieve developmental milestones. Accordingly, the age period described as adolescence may vary markedly from one individual to the next (Tanner, 1973).

Whilst the above difficulties in defining the adolescent period might appear academic, obvious practical difficulties may arise in the planning of services such as day-care or in-patient facilities for adolescent patients where arbitrary age limits need to be set. For example, an adolescent unit accepting youngsters between the ages of 12 and 17 may contain individual patients who are at very different stages of development (pre-pubertal, pubertal, or post-pubertal) and who consequently need to make quite different psychological adjustments. Such problems have given rise to the suggestion that placement should be made on biological rather than chronological grounds and that rigid age limits should be abolished (Court, 1976, paragraph 11.9 p. 166).

However, for the purpose of simplicity in this chapter the age period from 11 to 19 years will be considered.

## HEALTH NEEDS OF THE ADOLESCENT

In terms of physical illness, adolescents place far fewer demands upon the health service than younger children. Instead, the major health problems for adolescents lie within the social and behavioural sphere (Court, 1976). This fact presumably reflects the major developmental tasks of the adolescent period where the young person is striving to become independent from his or her family, beginning to form relationships with the opposite sex and also beginning to make major decisions about life ahead, for example in terms of education and employment. Traditionally adolescence has been viewed as a time of 'storm and stress' (Hall, 1904). Furthermore, some writers have suggested that a steady progress in development during this period is a sign of abnormality (Freud, 1952; Geleard, 1961). However, recent research has suggested that these views of adolescence may be misguided. Contrary to early speculation younger adolescents, at least, do not show increased evidence of psychological disturbance when compared with child or adult populations (Rutter *et al.*, 1976) nor do the *majority* of adolescents show the marked feelings of alienation and conflict with parents so often reported in literature (Douvan and Adelson, 1966; Bandura, 1972; Rutter *et al.*, 1976; Fogelman, 1976). Nevertheless, although some problems of adolescence are not necessarily more numerous than those of childhood in a number of respects they appear to differ in nature from those of earlier years. An example of this is that depression (Rutter *et al.*, 1976), suicide (Shaffer, 1974; Tyler, 1978), and attempted suicide (White, 1974) become more common in adolescence.

Other problems which have been reported to occur more frequently in adolescence are school refusal (Rutter *et al.*, 1970), anorexia nervosa (Crisp, 1967; Kendell *et al.*, 1973; Crisp *et al.*, 1976), drug dependence (Connell, 1976), and alcohol dependence (O'Connor, 1977). In addition, since in adolescence the young person is becoming sexually mature some problems (unwanted pregnancies, venereal disease, difficulty in sexual functioning) may occur as a result of this increased sexual activity (Schofield, 1973; Farrell, 1978). Finally, the incidence of some rarer psychiatric disorders such as schizophrenia (Rutter, 1972), manic depressive psychosis (Anthony and Scott, 1960), and obsessional compulsive states (Black, 1974) have been shown to increase in the adolescent period.

The wide ranging social and behavioural problems of adolescence described above bring young people into contact with many different agencies both within and outside the health service. For example, an adolescent who fails to attend school may be referred to the school psychological service, whilst another whose anxiety is expressed in physical symptoms may be referred to an appropriate hospital department for further investigation. Young people who break the law may have their first contacts with the police and juvenile courts. Subsequently they may be placed in care with the Local Authority and later maintained in a community home. Others with problems of drug addiction and fears of unwanted pregnancy who are afraid or unwilling to seek help through the family GP or hospital service may seek help from voluntary agencies. Youngsters whose parents are concerned about their behaviour may be taken to their general practitioner and subsequently referred to the child and adolescent psychiatric service; older adolescents may be referred to the adult psychiatric service. Table 10.1 lists some of the varied settings to which young people with psychological problems may be referred.

Traditionally, clinical psychologists specializing in adolescent problems have worked in psychiatric settings such as residential adolescent units. However, it is clear that any developing clinical psychology service for adolescents must establish close links with the wide network of agencies in health, education, and social services to which adolescents are referred.

TABLE 10.1 Settings to which adolescents with psychological problems may be referred

1. **Health**
   - (a) Health centres, general practice
   - (b) Hospital departments of child and adolescent psychiatry: out-patient, in-patient, and day-patient
   - (c) Hospital departments of adult psychiatry
   - (d) Other hospital departments, e.g. paediatrics, dermatology, wards admitting suicidal adolescents
   - (e) Child guidance clinics administered by NHS
   - (f) Special hospitals
   - (g) Youth treatment centres
2. **Education**
   - (a) Child guidance clinics administered by local authority departments
   - (b) Schools and units for maladjusted children (day and residential)
   - (c) Other special schools
3. **Social Services**
   - (a) Observation and assessment
   - (b) Community homes
   - (c) Community schools
4. **Voluntary Agencies**

   For example, Brook Advisory Centres, Grapevine Young People's Advisory Service, Samaritans

The progress that clinical psychologists have made in this direction is documented in the remaining sections of this chapter.

## DEVELOPMENT OF CLINICAL PSYCHOLOGY SERVICE FOR ADOLESCENTS

Although numbers of clinical psychologists in the health service have increased rapidly over the last 20 years (from 198 in 1962 to 795 in 1978 in England and Wales) the profession is still a relatively small one. Consequently the development of specialized services has only been possible in recent years. Nevertheless, individual clinical psychologists have been working with adolescents over quite a long period of time even though it has not been possible always to organize separate adolescent psychology services in the way envisaged by the Trethowan Report (1977).

It is difficult to trace the beginnings of this work with adolescents. However, unlike the educational psychology service which began independently with the appointment of the first local authority psychologist in 1913 and the establishment of the London Child Guidance Training Centre in 1928 the work of clinical psychologists with adolescents had its beginning in the establishment of child and adolescent psychiatric services within the NHS. The development of these services began following the National Health Service Act of 1946 which required the Regional Health Service Service Boards to provide medical services both in-patient and out-patient for children suffering from 'mental illness and maladjustment' (Howells, 1965). As new in-patient and day patient and out-patient facilities for adolescents were opened psychologists' posts were established to service these units.

In some cases posts were established to cover both child and adolescent services, in other cases posts were created specifically for work with adolescents, for example in adolescent in-patient units. By 1972 there were 257 beds for adolescents in such units and by 1974 — 436 beds (Court, 1976).

At the same time as these developments were taking place in the NHS demand for educational psychology services was also increasing. Following the Underwood Committee recommendation in 1955 educational psychologists were working in child guidance clinics and the school psychological service and these services provided an alternative source of help for disturbed adolescents. Furthermore, some older adolescents were being seen by clinical psychologists working in adult psychiatric settings and in the special hospitals.

However, during the 1970s a number of developments began to take place which led to a reappraisal of child and adolescent psychological services. The first of these was the reorganization of the health service which gave rise to increasing demands for the services of clinical psychologists.

A second development was the publishing of the Trethowan Report (DHSS, 1977) which recommended that clinical psychology services should be organized on an area basis and that individual psychologists should be made available to social service and education departments (para. 5.3.9). In addition, this report suggested that clinical psychologists should become more closely involved in primary care settings with general practitioners (para. 5.3.2).

The third influence was the Court Report published in 1976. This underlined the important role played by psychologists in the assessment and treatment of children and adolescents and recommended an expansion of the numbers of psychologists working in this field. Furthermore, it emphasized the advice giving role of psychologists to other professional workers.

Implicit in all these developments was the need for more extensive services. Clinical psychologists were being requested not only to see more children and adolescents but also to work in diverse settings (community homes, special schools, local authority hostels, community health centres). In addition they were being called upon to provide support for an increasing number of other professional groups including nurses, social workers, child care staff, and teachers.

From the results of a Division of Educational and Child Psychology (DECP) inquiry carried out in England and Wales (BPS, 1978a) it was clear that some of these influences were already having some impact on the work of clinical psychologists in health service settings. Tables 10.2 and 10.3 list some of the settings in which these psychologists were working together with the professionals with whom they had contact.

TABLE 10.2 Percentage of health service psychologists working in various settings with children and adolescents ($n = 91$)

| | | |
|---|---|---|
| 1. | Child Psychiatry Departments in hospitals | 86.6% |
| 2. | Paediatric Departments | 24.1% |
| 3. | Subnormality hospitals | 43.5% |
| 4. | Child Guidance Clinics | 22.9% |
| 5. | Special Day Schools | 19.0% |
| 6. | Community Health Centres | 13.2% |

Figures taken from 'Psychological services for children', *Bulletin of The British Psychological Society* (1978a) **31**, 11–15.

TABLE 10.3 Percentage of health service psychologists having contact with various professionals (at least monthly contact)

| | | |
|---|---|---|
| 1. | Psychiatrist | 85.0% |
| 2. | Other hospital doctors | 60.7% |
| 3. | Social services field workers | 52.3% |
| 4. | Teachers | 51.7% |
| 5. | Educational psychologists | 47.1% |
| 6. | Speech therapists | 39.0% |

Figures taken from 'Psychological services for children', *Bulletin of The British Psychological Society* (1978a) **31**, 11–15.

However, it was also clear that some of the recommendations of these reports could not be fully implemented. For example, the findings of the DECP inquiry that many of the NHS psychologists worked with children and adolescents through the age groups 0–19 years probably reflected the fact that in some localities there were too few psychologists to specialize solely in adolescent psychology services. This problem was met in some areas by one psychologist taking special responsibility for this service even though he/she was working with children of other age groups.

The DECP inquiry also showed that there was increasing liaison and co-operation between educational psychology and child psychology groups. However, with regard to the relationship between the two professional groups of psychologists the Court Report had made two controversial recommendations. First, this report suggested that the professions of educational and clinical psychology should be combined to form an integrated child psychology service. The second recommendation was that the distinction between child guidance clinics and child psychiatric hospital services should be dropped and that both should be reorganized as part of an integrated Child and Adolescent Psychiatry

Service. These suggestions were not met favourably by many educational and clinical psychologists and in 1978 the BPS voiced a number of objections to these recommendations in its comments to the Report (BPS, 1978b). As a result of some of these issues and the need for increasing co-operation between the two professional groups dealing with children and adolescents, the Professional Affairs Board of the BPS set up a working party to consider the future of psychological services for children and adolescents. At the time of going to press this body has still to make its final recommendations.

It is clear that clinical psychology services for adolescents are at an interesting stage of development. Although many areas are not yet able to support the specialized grouping of adolescent services headed by a principal psychologist envisaged by the Trethowan document the demand for such services exists. In the present economic climate a rapid expansion of services is obviously impossible. However, it is important to note that a number of psychologists have begun to extend their work with adolescents in a number of ways. For example, some have begun to work in association with social service departments or in community health settings. Moreover, some posts are being established which are jointly funded by health service and local authority. More detailed discussion of the role of a clinical psychologist in these settings will be left until the next section.

## THE ROLE OF THE CLINICAL PSYCHOLOGIST IN ADOLESCENT SERVICES

Traditionally in child and adolescent psychiatric services the psychologist was seen as having mainly an assessment function. For example, the psychologist's contribution to the multidisciplinary team would be to carry out psychometric assessment with the individual child or adolescent, whilst other workers would have the responsibility of assessing the family situation (Howells, 1965). However, in recent years a number of developments have effectively changed this rather limited role.

In the first instance, there has been substantial growth in the body of psychological knowledge concerning effective treatment methods. Moreover, in the last fifteen years or so psychologists have been responsible for the evolution of a number of sophisticated assessment procedures often involving direct observation of behaviour. These developments in assessment methods have enabled more detailed formulations of clinical problems to be made together with a closer monitoring of treatment progress. Inevitably this has led to an important role for psychologists in the treatment of adolescents.

Secondly, psychologists have become increasingly involved in indirect treatment methods by the transmission of their skills to other professional workers such as teachers, social workers, and child care staff. An examination of Table 10.4 shows that amongst all grades of child clinical psychologists below Principal level (field workers) the greatest proportion of time was spent in *indirect* treatment methods. Perhaps this has arisen partly from the impracticalities of

TABLE 10.4 Sessions worked by clinical psychologists in child and adolescent services on various categories of work

| Category of work | Principles (Full and part-time) ($N$ = 17) | | Field workers (Full and part-time) ($N$ = 66) | |
|---|---|---|---|---|
| | Mean no. of sessions | Per cent of total time | Mean no. of sessions | Per cent of total time |
| Direct treatment | 4.09 | 14.6 | 5.52 | 19.1 |
| Indirect treatment | 2.96 | 10.6 | 5.87 | 20.3 |
| Assessment, etc. | 5.08 | 18.1 | 5.31 | 18.4 |
| Planning | 3.89 | 13.9 | 2.71 | 9.4 |
| Administration | 2.41 | 8.6 | 2.42 | 8.4 |
| Data collection | 2.44 | 8.7 | 1.14 | 3.9 |
| Professional development | 2.41 | 8.6 | 1.57 | 5.4 |
| Training | 3.57 | 12.7 | 3.10 | 10.7 |
| Other | 1.18 | 4.2 | 1.23 | 4.3 |
| Total | 28.03 | 100.0 | 28.87 | 100.0 |

Figures taken from *Psychological Services for Children in England and Wales*, DECP (1980).

carrying out individual treatment in the face of increasing demand for psychological services and partly from a growing emphasis on the interactive nature of the problems of children and adolescents.

A third development arises from the involvement of some psychologists in the wider aspects of the policy and planning of treatment environments.

## TREATMENT WITH INDIVIDUALS

It is impossible in the limited space available to give a detailed account of treatment methodologies with adolescent youngsters. However, it is possible to draw attention to some issues underlying therapy and to illustrate these by specific examples.

Adolescent problems are of a multifactorial nature. Accordingly, different factors may produce and maintain the *same* problem behaviour in different youngsters. For this reason it is not possible to apply psychological treatments to a particular problem in a 'cookbook fashion'. Many psychologists adopt what has been termed an 'applied scientist' approach to clinical problems (Davidson, 1977). Fundamental to this approach is (1) a careful and objective description of the problem, (2) a detailed formulation of the problem (that is setting up hypotheses concerning the origins and maintenance of the problem), and (3) a systematic testing of the hypotheses through treatment inverventions, the effects of which are closely monitored.

One of the important stages in this process is the formulation of the clinical problem. It is often tempting in clinical practice, when a presenting problem is one for which effective treatment methods have been found, to embark upon treatment without an adequate clinical formulation. However such a short cut may be misguided. A practical example of this issue arose in an out-patient clinic held by the author to which a sixteen-year-old boy was referred with problems of obsessional handwashing and cleaning rituals. These rituals had persisted for several months and were taking up much of the young man's time so that he was in danger of losing his job as a lorry driver's mate. He was extremely reluctant to talk about his problems but clearly was very distressed so that it was tempting to embark upon a programme involving response prevention (Meyer *et al*., 1974) and flooding (Marks *et al*., 1975) as quickly as possible. However, a detailed analysis of the problem over a number of sessions revealed that the young man had been experiencing a great deal of anxiety concerning his first experiences of sexual attraction towards a young woman staying in his parent's home. His high level of anxiety had given rise to a number of physical symptoms including increased frequency of urination which he had interpreted as a sign of venereal disease. His excessive handwashing and cleanliness was an attempt to protect his family from his 'infection' and was maintained by anxiety reduction. He had had no sexual experience and his knowledge concerning sex was extremely limited. Figure 1 gives a simple formulation of the problem. This anecdotal example illustrates how a premature programme using response prevention and flooding would have been both time consuming and costly. In this case rapid progress was achieved and complete elimination of the compulsive handwashing within three sessions which focused upon (a) an explanation of his physical symptoms; (b) factual information concerning sexual functioning and sexual relationships.

A similar emphasis on the detailed formulation of clinical problems has been given by Slade (1982) in the case of adolescent anorexic behaviour. In this model the eating problem of the anorexic patient is viewed not as the primary disorder but as a 'secondary adaptation to a more general set of psychological problems'. Using this formulation one of the most important goals of treatment is to enable the anorexic girl to establish sources of satisfaction other than dieting. Accordingly this view would support the notion expressed by some writers of the misguided nature of treatment methods which have placed central attention on weight gain as the main goal in therapy for anorexic patients (Bemis, 1978).

The wide ranging problems of adolescents include anxiety, depression, difficulties in interpersonal relationships, delinquent behaviour, sexual problems, drug taking, heavy drinking, and attempted suicide. These problems differ in nature from those of childhood and reflect some of the developmental tasks of the adolescent period. Undoubtedly one of the major tasks for the adolescent is to gain independence from the family. However, some young people may suffer considerable anxiety in taking steps towards independence whilst others may find that their independent actions bring them in conflict with the police or

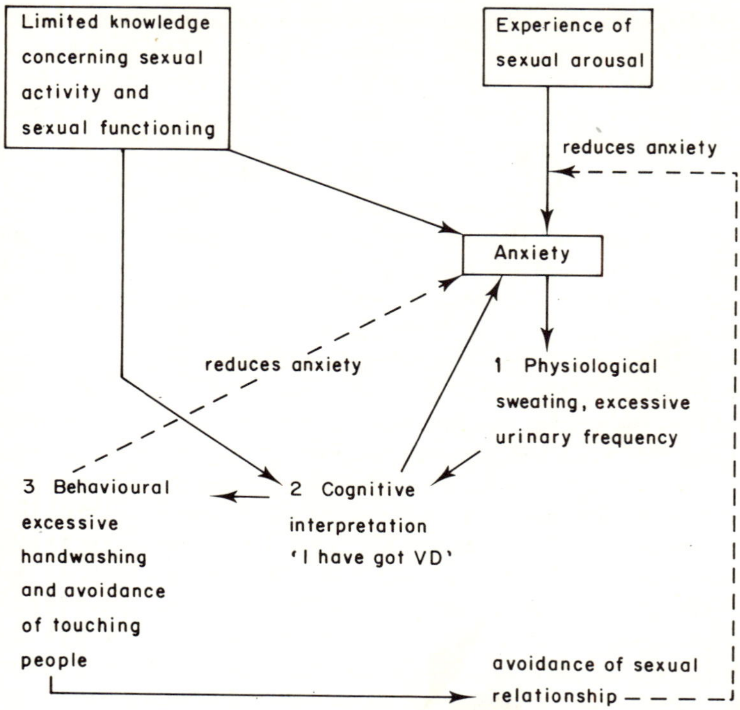


FIG. 1 Clinical formulation of obsessional handwashing in a 16-year-old male adolescent

school authorities. A fundamental aim of therapy then is to aid the young person to gain independence by developing their problem solving skills in a way that will allow them to avoid undue psychological distress.

Such an approach was adopted by Yule and his colleagues (Yule *et al.*, 1980) in behavioural treatment of a twelve-year-old boy with school refusal problems which had developed following a period of ill-health and a subsequent hospitalization. Significant factors were fears of academic failure linked to high academic goals, decreased performance at school prior to school refusal due to high anxiety and loss of concentration, later phobic avoidance of school and school friends and specific anxiety associated with inability to explain his absence to school friends. Successful treatment involved increasing the youngster's coping strategies by training in relaxation skills, graded exposure in imagination and in real-life, lowering in academic goals (moving into a lower stream at school), rehearsal and role-playing to enable him to explain his absence to his school friends. Similar approaches to the treatment of school phobia have been described by psychologists working in educational settings (Blagg, 1977; Galloway, 1980).

A second example of treatment as a training in problem solving skills arises in the treatment of young offenders. It has been argued that delinquent behaviour of some youngsters arises because the young person has not learnt appropriate ways of responding in some social situations. A youngster may, for example, use aggressive behaviour to obtain a desired goal in the absence of any other alternative behavioural strategy. An interesting approach to treatment of delinquent behaviour has been developed by a number of psychologists who have been carrying out social skills training programmes with young offenders in a community home setting. Such programmes have included training in a range of skills from quite specific behaviours such as eye contact and head movements (Spence and Marzillier, 1979) to more complex interaction skills such as interviewing techniques, dealing with teasing, bullying and criticism (Spence and Spence, 1980). Similar studies in the USA have used social skills training procedures to train the predelinquent adolescent and their families in negotiation skills to avoid family conflict (Kifer *et al.*, 1974) whilst others working with unemployed adolescents have specifically trained young people in job finding skills (Azrin *et al.*, 1975). A number of writers have noted the association between low self-esteem and delinquency (Eitzen, 1975; Herbert, 1978). In this regard it is interesting to note that youngsters undergoing social skills training described above showed increases in self-esteem on pre- and post-treatment questionnaires (Spence and Spence, 1980). Although these changes were shortlived and had disappeared by a six-month follow-up, it is important to note that such changes in self-esteem can occur with minimal treatment intervention, in this case one hour group sessions.

## INDIRECT TREATMENT

An important aspect of the changing role of the clinical psychologist is the use of indirect treatment methods involving transmission of skills to parents, nurses, teachers and child care staff. Particularly influential in this respect are the writings of some American psychologists (Tharp and Wetzel, 1969; Patterson, 1974). In this country examples of this approach are to be found within social service settings. For instance, one group of workers have investigated the feasibility of the implementation of a behavioural treatment programme for enuresis by child care staff within a community home setting. The incidence of bed wetting is reported to be particularly high amongst children in residential homes (Stein and Susser, 1967; Yule and Raynes, 1972). Moreover, such a problem may impose considerable restrictions on fostering or return to parents. There are obvious advantages of finding a successful treatment method for enuretic youngsters living in such residential settings.

A group of 39 children in 34 children's homes took part in the study; 19 in a treatment group and a further 20 in a no-treatment control group. The children's homes ranged from small family units to larger residential establishments. Most children slept in dormitories and only one of the children had his own room. Treatment involved the regular use of an enuresis alarm over a number of weeks. The alarm consists of two metal gauze detector pads which are assembled on the bed at night and connected to an alarm box which is placed at the side of the bed. Urination during the night causes the alarm to ring and the child to awaken. Although this form of treatment is extremely successful in out-patient settings (see, for example, Taylor and Turner, 1975) difficulties could clearly arise in community homes where there are a multiplicity of staff caring for children and where other children in a dormitory could easily be disturbed. The study, therefore, set out to examine the effectiveness and the feasibility of carrying out this treatment programme within a community home setting (Jehu *et al.*, 1977).

To ensure adequate compliance with treatment instructions house-parents were asked to make sure that youngsters got up and went to the toilet when the alarm sounded. They were also asked to help remake the bed, reset the alarm, and keep a record of wet and dry nights.

As a result of treatment all but one of the children in the treatment group ceased to wet the bed at night whereas youngsters in the control group did not improve significantly. The mean duration of treatment was 12 weeks. It is interesting to note that some youngsters were also reported to have improved more generally in their behaviour. Moreover, staff reported minimal disruption in the homes and expressed an enthusiasm to use the treatment method again with other enuretic children.

Such a study clearly indicated one way that psychologists might usefully provide a behaviourally oriented support service to help residential staff in the management of children with difficult behaviour problems. Another example arises from the social skills training programme described earlier where attempts are now being made to involve child care staff in the teaching of social skills to youngsters in community schools (Spence and Marzillier, 1979).

Psychologists have also been involved in a consultant role in other aspects of social service work. For example, a number of local authorities have been operating family placement schemes for children who would otherwise be placed in a community home school (Hazel and Cox, 1976). In Birmingham some psychologists have been involved in giving advice to foster parents on how to deal with problems of management of these sometimes difficult youngsters (Druce, 1977).

More extensive examples of this approach can be seen in those units that have adopted a social learning theory philosophy such that the whole unit is run along behavioural lines. One psychologist has described the setting up of such a regime within Youth Treatment Centres (YTC) (Reid, 1981). YTCs are units which were initially set up to provide special long term treatment facilities for disturbed adolescents who could not easily be contained within the community home system and youngsters who had committed serious offences and were detained under Section 53 of the Children and Young Peoples Act, 1933 (Cawson and Martell, 1975). There are now two such units in the country, the units are under the direct control of the DHSS and act as an extension to the secure units already providing for difficult boys within the community homes system.

Reid (1981) has listed some of the problem behaviours of the young people referred to these units. As can be seen in Table 10.5 these behaviours are wide ranging and provide a sizeable problem for any institution attempting to provide a comprehensive treatment programme.

TABLE 10.5 Problem behaviours of young people referred to a Youth Treatment Centre (from Reid, 1981)

1. **Major offence behaviours**
   - Murder
   - Manslaughter
   - Armed robbery
   - Sexual assaults
   - Arson

2. **Minor offence behaviours**
   - Theft
   - Take and drive away
   - Burglary
   - Prostitution

3. **'Clinical' problems**
   - Obsessional rituals (e.g. washing, dressing, thoughts)
   - Enuresis
   - Faecal smearing
   - Anxiety

4. **Behavioural deficits**
   - Limited intellectual ability
   - Lack of educational attainment
   - Lack of social skills (verbal and non-verbal)
   - Lack of survival skills (e.g. self-help budgeting, etc.)

5. **Behavioural excesses**
   - Physical violence (persons and property)
   - Self-mutilation (head banging, wrist slashing, overdoses)
   - Verbal violence

6. **Institutional problem behaviours**
   - Hostages
   - Sit in/barricades
   - Sexual behaviour
   - Violence
   - Attempted escapes

7. **Problems of generalization**
   - Self-help skills
   - Job skills – interview behaviour, work skills, etc.
   - Family conflicts
   - Deviant peer group
   - Abscondings

In Glenthorne Youth Treatment Centre the clinical psychologists act mainly in an advisory capacity whilst the 'front-line' therapists are group workers coming from the teaching, nursing, and child care professions.

The main goal of treatment is to establish through reinforcement, modelling, and instruction, behavioural competence in social, educational, vocational, and self-care skills. In addition, attempts are made to modify those disruptive behaviours that have often brought youngsters to the centre in the first instance.

Initially, all young people entering the YTC are admitted into the assessment unit which is run as a points economy system. Here young people earn points for achieving specified goals. Accordingly, this unit allows a detailed assessment to be made of the youngsters' level of functioning. From here allocation is made either to one of the secure units or to an open unit or hostel. As the youngster progresses to lessening degrees of security, fewer prompts are given by staff and more reliance is given to naturally occurring contingencies (e.g. verbal approval, self-control). In addition, youngsters are able to spend increasing amounts of time outside the centre and practise developing skills in the 'real world'. Great emphasis is placed on the flexible design of individual programmes, direct observation, and detailed monitoring of achievement goals by staff (Reid, 1981).

Although this centre is in its early stages of development the treatment approach which emphasizes the acquisition of positive problem solving skills appears to be extremely promising.

## POLICY AND PLANNING

In an article concerning the development of 'community psychology' one psychologist has described the importance of a multilevel approach within clinical psychology services. Three levels are described: (1) working with clients individually or in groups; (2) working with staff in order to help larger groups of clients; and (3) working with managers in monitoring policy and planning (Bender, 1979). The involvement of some psychologists in the setting up of total treatment environments has given rise to their participation in the policy and planning of such institutions (Brown, 1977; Brown and Sawyer, 1978; Reid, 1981). For example in the YTC described earlier the principal psychologist has become the Programme Director with a line management function and responsibility for the overall treatment programme of the institution, staff recruitment, and staff training (Fig. 10.2). An important part of this new role for psychologists is the undertaking of careful research investigations into the effectiveness of different types of policy and provision for young people (see, for example, Cornish and Clarke, 1975). Such studies provide a firm factual basis upon which policy and planning decisions can be made.

## FUTURE PROGRESS OF CLINICAL PSYCHOLOGY SERVICES FOR ADOLESCENTS

Previous sections have outlined some of the psychological needs of adolescents and have pointed to some of the contributions of clinical psychologists working in different health and social service settings. It is clear that although psychological services for adolescents are at an early stage of development there is considerable potential for increasing the application of psychological skills and knowledge in this field. It is worthwhile in this concluding section, therefore, to consider avenues for future development of the service.

(1) The high rates of suicidal behaviour in adolescents are well known (Morgan *et al.*, 1975; Tyler, 1978). Many adolescents make repeated attempts at taking their own lives. Furthermore, some young people learn that this behaviour is one effective, if drastic, way of obtaining help. At least one study has noted that once referred such children take up quite a large proportion of

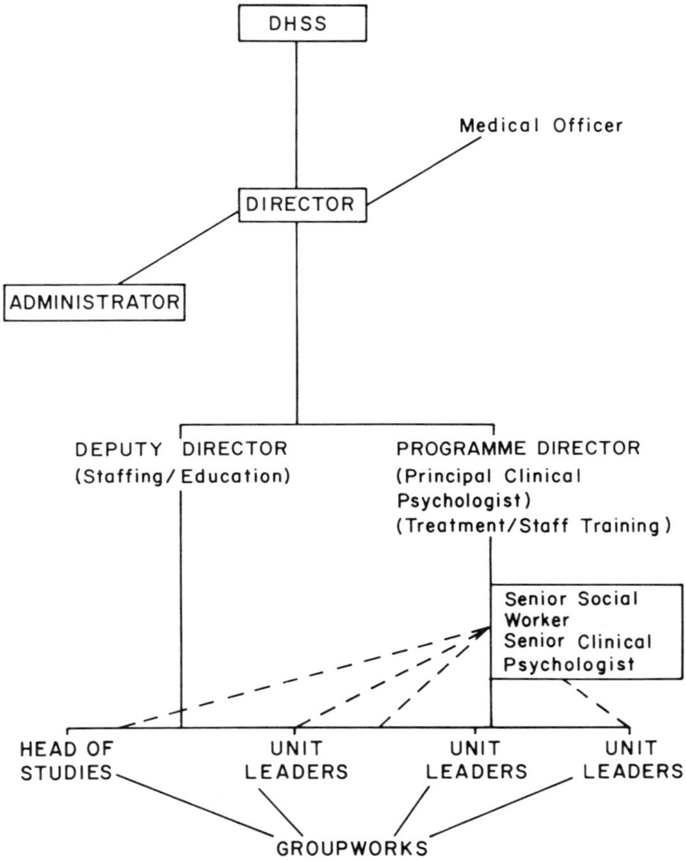


FIG. 2 Glenthorne Youth Treatment Centre

psychiatric services, since they are more likely to be admitted into hospital, once in hospital they are more likely to remain there for longer and once discharged they are more likely to be sent for further institutional care or treatment than children referred with other problems (Mattson *et al.*, 1969). Suicide and depressive behaviour in young people becomes therefore one of the major health concerns of the adolescent population.

Close liaison with casualty departments and early intervention through the establishment of crisis counselling services may enable psychological services to prevent the repetitive cycle of suicide attempts and psychiatric hospital admission for some of these young people. In particular utilization of cognitive behaviour therapy methods currently proving useful in the treatment of depression in adult populations (Blackburn *et al.*, 1981) may equip young people with strategies which would enable them to deal more effectively with future depressive episodes.

(2) No mention has been made in the earlier sections of this chapter of the effects of physical illness on young people. In the USA some psychologists have established counselling services for such patients and for the terminally ill. One counselling service for terminally ill adolescents was set up recently in this country (Kuykendall, 1981). Preliminary investigations in Liverpool (Edwards, 1982) suggest that this may be a useful area for future development. This type of counselling service for adolescents with serious illnesses and for their parents could well be offered as part of an adolescent clinical psychology service.

(3) Reference was made earlier to the number of young women who face unwanted pregnancies. Although overall rates for illegitimate birth and abortions in young women (11 – 19 years) have stabilized in recent years, the number of abortions to younger adolescents (11 – 15 years) has continued to rise (Court, 1976). In this respect it is interesting to note that a recent article commenting on the clinical psychology servicing of an obstetrics and gynaecology department paid particular attention to the need for termination counselling for young girls in this setting (Broome, 1980).

(4) As many young people find it easier to seek help from bodies not associated with home or school, a fourth potential area for liaison work exists in the field of voluntary services. Clinical psychologists specializing in the psychological treatment of sexual problems, problem drinking, and drug addiction may well be able to offer a specialist support service in such settings.

(5) Finally, many clinical psychologists have already established close links with GPs and community health centres. Such developments are also important for adolescent services where early identification of psychological problems may prevent compulsory hospitalization at a later stage. In such setting some psychologists have established self-help groups for young people (for eating problems, see Caswell, 1976) whilst others have become involved in the use of family therapy (for reviews, see Minuchin, 1974; Skynner, 1976). Clearly this type of service could well extend in the future.

However, it is perhaps important to add a few cautionary remarks to the above suggestions for the future development of clinical psychology services for adolescents. In the first place, as noted earlier, problems of adolescents are wide ranging, encompassing difficulties within the social, psychological, vocational, and medical domains. Youngsters may have problems adapting in the family, in the school, or at work and these problems may bring the young person into contact with many different professional agencies. Any development of clinical psychology services must take into account the provision made by other agencies for adolescent problems and clear links should be developed both at the level of policy and planning and at a more personal level between one professional and another.

Secondly, it is not sufficient simply to demonstrate that there is a need for increased services and then to supply that need. The establishment of new services should be closely monitored and their effectiveness ascertained. Furthermore, there is an overriding need for more research into adolescent problems, a fact that was noted recently by the SSRC by the establishment of a special fund to promote research in this area (Schaffer and Hargreaves, 1978).

In a number of ways the problems of adolescents have been neglected in health service provision. The setting up of more effective services for both prevention and treatment may ensure the avoidance of later crises in adult life.

## REFERENCES

Anthony, J., and Scott, P. (1960). Manic-depressive psychosis in childhood. *Journal of Child Psychology and Psychiatry,* **1**, 53–72.

Azrin, N. H., Flores, T., and Kaplan, S. J. (1975). Job finding club: A group assisted programme for obtaining employment. *Behaviour Research and Therapy,* **13**, 17–28.

Bandura, A. (1972). The stormy decade: Fact or fiction? In D. Rogers (ed.) *Issues in Adolescent Psychology*, 2nd ed. New York: Appleton-Century-Crofts.

Bemis, K. (1978). Current approaches to the etiology and treatment of anorexia nervosa. *Psychological Bulletin,* **85**, 593–617.

Bender, M. P. (1979). Community psychology: When? *Bulletin of The British Psychological Society,* **32**, 6–9.

Black, A. (1974). The natural history of obsessional neurosis. In R. Beech (ed.) *Obsessional States.* London: Methuen.

Blackburn, I. M., Bishop, S., Glen, A. I. M., Whalley, L., and Christie, J. C. (1981). The efficacy of cognitive therapy in depression: A treatment trial using cognitive therapy and pharmcotherapy, each alone and in combination. *British Journal of Psychiatry,* **139**, 181–189.

Blagg, N. (1977). A detailed strategy for the rapid treatment of school phobics. *British Association of Behavioural Psychotherapy Bulletin,* **5**, 70–75.

British Psychological Society (1978a). Psychological services for children. *Bulletin of The British Psychological Society,* **31**, 125–127.

British Psychological Society (1978b). The Society's comments on the Report of the Court Committee on Child Health Services. *Bulletin of The British Psychological Society,* **31**, 157–160.

Broome, A. K. (1980). Clinical psychology within obstetrics and gynaecology. *Bulletin of The British Psychological Society,* **33**, 357–359.

Brown, B. (1977). Gillbey House: A token economy management scheme in a residential school for adolescent boys in trouble. *British Association of Behavioural Psychotherapy,* **5**, 79–89.

Brown, B. J. and Sawyer, C. E. (1978). Uses and abuses of psychologists — Some alternatives for psychologists working in social services departments. *Bulletin of the British Psychological Society,* **31**, 218–222.

Caswell, G. (1976). A study to compare the effectiveness of the behavioural modification of eating habits with dietary advice to overweight adolescent girls. Unpublished M.Sc. Thesis, Leeds.

Cawson, P., and Martell, P. (1975). Children referred to closed units. DHSS Research Report No. 5. London: HMSO.

Coleman, J. C. (1980). *The Nature of Adolescence.* New York: Methuen.

Connell, P. (1976). Clinical aspects of drug misuse. In M. Rutter and L. Hersov (eds), *Child Psychiatry: Modern Approaches.* Oxford: Blackwell Scientific Publications.

Cornish, D. B., and Clarke, R. V. G. (1975). Residential treatment and its effects on delinquency. London: HMSO.

Court, S. D. M. (1976). *Fit for the future: The report of the Committee on Child Health Services.* London: HMSO.

Crisp, A. H. (1965). Some aspects of the evolution presentation and follow-up of anorexia nervosa. *Procedings of The Royal Society of Medicine,* **58**, 814–820.
Crisp, A. H. (1967). Anorexia nervosa. *Hospital Medicine,* **I**, 713–718.
Crisp. A. H., Palmer, R. L., and Kallucy, R. S. (1976). How common is anorexia nervosa? *British Journal of Psychiatry,* **128**, 549–554.
Davidson, M. (1977). The scientific/applied debate in psychology: A contribution. *Bulletin of The British Psychological Society,* **30**, 273–278.
Division of Educational and Clinical Psychology (1978). Psychological services for children. *Bulletin of The British Psychological Society,* **31**, 11–15.
Douvan, E., and Adelson, J. (1966). *The Adolescent Experience.* New York: Wiley.
Druce, N. R. (1977). Social learning approaches to professional fostering and treatment with security. In Behavioural Approaches to the Treatment of Delinquent Adolescents. Unpublished manuscript: Tennal School.
Edwards, G. (1982). A study of adjustment and illness related anxieties in adolescents with cystic fibrosis in relation to communication and denial within the family. Unpublished M. Psychol. dissertation, University of Liverpool.
Eitzen, D. S. (1975). The effects of behaviour modification on the attitude of delinquents. *Behaviour Research and Therapy,* **13**, 295–299.
Farrell, C. (1978). *My Mother Said.* London: Routledge and Kegan Paul.
Fogelman, K. (1976). *Britain's Sixteen Year Olds.* London: National Children's Bureau.
Freud, A. (1952). Adolescence. *Psychoanalytic Study of the Child,* **13**, 255–278.
Galloway, D. (1980). Problems in the assessment and management of persistent absenteeism from school. In L. Hersov and I. Berg (eds). *Out of School.* Chichester: Wiley.
Geleard, E. R. (1961). Some aspects of ego vicissitudes in adolescence. *Journal of The American Psychoanalytic Association,* **9**, 394–350.
Graham, P. and Rutter, M. (1976). Adolescent disorders. In M. Rutter and L. Hersov (eds) *Child Psychiatry: Modern Approaches.* Oxford: Blackwell Scientific Publications.
Hall, G. S. (1904). *Adolescence, its Psychology and its Relations to Psychology, Anthropology, Sociology, Sex, Crime, Religion and Education*, Vols. I and II. New York: Appleton.
Hazel, N., and Cox, R. (1976). First report of the Special Family Project. Kent Social Services Department.
Herbert, M. (1978). *Conduct Disorders of Childhood and Adolescence: A Behavioural Approach to Assessment and Treatment.* Chichester: Wiley.
Howells, J. (1965). Organisation of child psychiatric services. In G. Howell (ed.), *Modern Perspectives in Adolescent Psychiatry*. Edinburgh: Oliver and Boyd.
Jehu, D., Morgan, R. T. T., Turner, R., and Jones, A. (1977). A controlled trial of the treatment of nocturnal enuresis in residential homes for children. *Behavioural Research and Therapy,* **15**, 1–16.
Kendell, R. E., Hall, D. J., Hailey, A., and Babigian, H. M. (1973). The epidemiology of anorexia nervosa. *Psychological Medicine,* **3**, 200–203.
Kennedy, P., Krietman, N., and Ovenstone, I. (1974). The prevalence of suicide and parasuicide (attempted suicide) in Edinburgh. *British Journal of Psychiatry,* **124**, 36–41.
Kifer, R. E., Lewis, M. A., Green, D. R., and Phillips, E. L. (1974). Training predelinquent youths and their parents to negotiate conflict situations. *Journal of Applied Behaviour Analysis,* **7**, 357–364.
Kuykendall, J. (1981). Personal communication.
Marks, I. M., Hodgson, R., and Rachman, S. (1975). Treatment of chronic obsessive-compulsive neurosis by in vivo exposure. *British Journal of Psychiatry,* **127**, 349–364.
Meyer, V., Levy, R., and Schnurer, A. (1974). The behavioural treatment of obsessive

compulsive disorders. In H. R. Beech (ed.), *Obsessional States*. London: Methuen.
Mattson, A., Seese, L. R., and Hawkins, J. W. (1969). Suicidal behaviour as a child psychiatric emergency. *Archives of General Psychiatry,* **20**, 100–109.
Minuchin, S. (1974). *Families and Family Therapy*. London: Tavistock.
Morgan, H. G., Pocock, H., and Pottle, S. (1975). The urban distribution of non-fatal deliberate self-harm. *British Journal of Psychiatry*, **126**, 319–328.
O'Connor, J. (1977). Normal and problem drinking among children. *Journal of Child Psychology and Psychiatry,* **18**, 279–284.
Patterson, G. R. (1974). Interventions with boys with conduct problems: Multiple settings, treatments and criteria. *Journal of Consulting Psychology,* **42**, 471–481.
Reid, I. (1981). The development and maintenance of a behavioural regime in a secure treatment centre. In M. P. Feldman (ed.) *Development in the Study of Criminal Behaviour, Volume I: The Prevention and Control of Offenders*. London: Wiley.
Rutter, M. (1972). Childhood schizophrenia reconsidered. *Journal of Autism and Schizophrenia,* **2**, 315–337.
Rutter, M., Graham, P., Chadwick, O., and Yule, W. (1976). Adolescent turmoil: Fact or fiction. *Journal of Child Psychology and Psychiatry,* **17**, 35–56.
Rutter, M., Tizard, J., and Whitmore, K. (1970). *Education, Health and Behaviour*. London: Longman.
Schaffer, H. R., and Hargreaves, D. (1978). Young people in the society: A research initiative by the SSRC. *Bulletin of The British Psychological Society,* **31**, 81–94.
Schofield, M. (1965). *The Sexual Behaviour of Young People*. London: Longman.
Schofield, M. (1973). *The Sexual Behaviour of Young Adults*. London: Allen Lane.
Shaffer, D. (1974). Suicide in Childhood and Early Adolescence. *Journal of Child Psychology and Psychiatry,* **15**, 275–291.
Shaw, C., and Shelkun, R. (1965). Suicidal adolescents and children. *Psychiatry,* **28**, 157–168.
Skynner, R. (1976). *One Flesh Separate Persons*. London: Constable.
Slade, P. (1982). Towards a functional analysis of anorexia and bulimia nervosa. *British Journal of Clinical Psychology*, **21**, 167–179.
Spence, S. H., and Marzillier, J. (1979). Social skills training with adolescent male offenders: I — short term effects. *Behavioural Research and Therapy,* **17**, 7–16.
Spence, A. J. and Spence S. H. (1980). Cognitive changes associated with social skills training. *Behaviour Research and Therapy*, **18**, 265–272.
Stein, Z. A., and Susser, M. (1967). The social dimensions of a symptom: A socio-medical study of enuresis. *Social Science and Medicine,* **1**, 183–201.
Tanner, J. M. (1973). *Growing-Up. Scientific American,* **229**, 35–42.
Taylor, P. D., and Turner, R. K. (1975). A clinical trial of continuous intermittent and overlearning 'bell and pad' treatments for nocturnal enuresis. *Behavioural Research and Therapy,* **13**, 281–293.
Tharp, R. C., and Wetzel, R. J. (1969). *Behaviour Modification in the Natural Environment*. New York: Academic Press.
Trethowan, W. H. (1977). *The Role of Psychologists in the Health Services*. London: HMSO.
Tyler, M. (1978). Advisory and counselling services for young people. DHSS Research Report No. 1. London: HMSO.
White, H. C. (1974). Self poisoning in adolescents. *British Journal of Psychiatry,* **124**, 24–35.
Yule, W., Hersov, L., and Treseder, J. (1980). Behavioural treatments in school refusal. In L. Hersov and I. Berg (eds) *Out of School*. Chichester: Wiley.
Yule, W., and Raynes, N. V. (1972). Behavioural characteristics of children in residential care in relation to indices of separation. *Journal of Child Psychology and Psychiatry,* **13**, 249–258.

The Practice of Clinical Psychology in Great Britain
Edited by A. Liddell


# *Chapter 11*

# *Psychological services for the elderly*

*Peter G. Britton*

The early 1980s will see an increase in the impact of an ageing population on most developed countries. There has been a dramatic rise in the numbers of those surviving to over seventy-five years of age in the last fifty years. Current projections envisage some 20 per cent of the population in the late twentieth century being over sixty-five with an increasing build-up of the very old (over eighty). This group of clients will provide a continuing challenge for the helping professions as the emphasis changes from keeping people alive to ensuring that the quality of life is maintained into old age. Psychology has much to offer in this area.

As we explore the impact of the needs of the elderly it is interesting to note the attitudes of potential clinical psychologists to work in this area. In a survey of applicants for training in clinical psychology (Liddell and Boyle, 1980), the prospect of work with the elderly did not seem at all appealing, indeed, it was among the lowest rated areas. Obviously, there is a need for some effective communication of the potential for significant change which the involvement of modern psychology can bring.

We will explore the scope of the work of psychologists in relation to the older client and attempt to evaluate current approaches. It is relevant that the past few years have seen the emergence of interest groupings of psychologists concerned with the care of the elderly in the United Kingdom. Such a development gives an indication that the involvement of psychologists has moved from the work of a few pioneers into a more stable phase of evolution. This should greatly assist in the dissemination of knowledge of the potential of psychology for this group and in an improvement of impact and image.

Despite the inevitability of ageing and of its impact upon society there was little evidence of much systematic study of the psychological processes involved in the early part of the century. However, the economic recession of the 1930s provoked interest in problems associated with the ageing process. Many workers in middle or old age were thrown out of employment and in their subsequent retraining and adjustment it was realized that far too little was known about the underlying psychological process of ageing. The work of

Miles at Stanford in the first major research unit on the psychology of ageing in this era provided a foundation for much later work. The importance of a multidisciplinary approach was soon recognized and continues to date. A re-examination of the work of the psychologists of this period is enlightening as we today face similar problems of economic recession and technological change.

The years since 1945 have seen an upsurge of interest in the study of the ageing and aged. The Nuffield Unit at Cambridge, set up by Bartlett and associated with the books by Welford (1951, 1958) on *Skill and Age*, carried out work on the ageing process which had a significant impact and is still highly relevant. On the clinical side the work of Martin Roth and his associates at Newcastle provided from 1955 an increasing awareness of the incidence of mental disorder in old age and its psychological consequences. In the USA long-term studies at the University of Chicago under Havinghurst and the Duke University project under Buss have made a significant contribution. These projects have provided longitudinal data on both general measures and trends in ageing and on very specific processes.

In recent years research has been considerably assisted by advances in knowledge of the methodology relevant to age-related change. The work of Schaie (1965 *et seq.*) deserves particular mention in drawing attention to the necessity for appropriate methodology to avoid the many traps of inference which exist in this area.

As psychology and in particular clinical psychology has expanded from an interest in the definition of behaviour to intervention, a similar trend has been seen in relation to ageing research. The 1970s have seen a move into the application to the elderly of a wide variety of psychological treatment techniques which have been found to be as relevant to this age group as to many others. Perhaps, the fundamental change has been from an acceptance of the common myth of seemingly inevitable deterioration, towards an approach which seeks out and reinforces the positive and adaptive aspects of behaviour.

The remainder of this chapter will attempt to explore some aspects of the current situation. We will first concentrate on the contribution of the psychologist to late middle age and the retirement phase, and look then at stable old age with a final examination of some problems which are liable to occur in the aged.

## PREPARATION FOR AGEING AND OLD AGE

Despite the inevitability of ageing there has been a marked reluctance actively to prepare people for the changes which may occur in the later phases of working life, through retirement to old age. In the past ten years economic changes have consistently eroded the previously clear distinction between 'working life' and 'retirement'. A combination of economic and technological factors has produced an indistinct phase of adjustment which may occur at any point in the 40 to 60 age range. Retirement has taken on a new and broader meaning (Council of Europe, 1977).

Education of those involved in this period of adjustment is clearly essential. There are many myths and misconceptions about the older worker. A typical example is that of an excessive behavioural rigidity, a resistance to change or inability to compensate. However, the studies of the older worker carried out by a variety of psychologists over the years suggest a more positive approach. Provided that retraining is appropriate, with attention paid to factors such as subdivision of skills to basic components, initial overlearning and appropriate reinforcement, the older worker *can* adapt. Indeed, if one takes motivation into account the determination to succeed can be far higher than in those who are younger.

Some problems remain, particularly for the worker who finds a rapidly changing job situation as his adaptive ability lessens. On the one hand compensation may occur, for example the automatic lathe capitalizes on the skill and experience of the older worker to set it up, then performs the repetitive work itself. On the other hand change may be hard to accept in other skilled tasks such as those of the compositor in a printing works who faces a non-repetitive task with severe memory load and requiring perceptual motor-skills of a high level. However, even in this case technology is again providing new methods such as computer typesetting which can make the impact of ageing less acute.

Life satisfaction for the individual moving into retirement involves much more than the work situation. The influences of family and home environment must be taken into account. As the age of retirement reduces it is likely that it will increasingly concentrate the psychological impact of other significant life events, such as the movement of children from the nuclear family on marriage, and the death of parents, into a smaller age span. This is likely to have cumulative stress effects which may require specialized counselling.

As we have previously stated, preparation for the changes in this phase to encourage positive adaptation seems crucial. The topic has been approached in a variety of ways ranging from formal 'Preparation for Retirement Courses' such as those mounted by the Glasgow Retirement Council to informal education provided by interest groups. Such help is currently available only to a very small proportion of those in need. Only rarely do individuals at this stage actively seek help from psychologists or social workers.

Such courses may include information on the medical, psychiatric, financial, and social aspects of age change and within the psychological and behavioural area cover a broad range of topics. These may include ideas of expected changes in intellect, personality, and adjustment and advice on coping with continuing demands for such diverse skills as social and sexual behaviour.

The necessity for adequate preparation for the retirement process and the broader changes associated with adjustment from middle to old age seems well proven. There is an obvious need for more specific psychological research and resource provision in this area. An attempt should be made to evaluate the relation between the provision of information and later adjustment. However, it may be assumed that the common fears of becoming old are often unnecessarily reinforced by a total ignorance of what might be realistically expected.

## STABLE OLD AGE

Once the problems of a change in role at retirement have been overcome the ageing person can reasonably expect a period of relatively active and productive life. There are obvious consequences of the varied but inevitable changes in physical ability with increasing age. Changes in the locomotor, cardiovascular, and respiratory systems are likely to impose increasing restrictions on activity. However, unless these occur in combination, maintenance of a level of activity conducive to reasonable adjustment is usually possible.

On the psychological side there are some interesting ideas to explore. An unfortunate and fairly general misconception is that general intellectual abilities suffer a significant and inevitable decline after the age of sixty. Psychological research in the past decade has shown that this is not a reasonable assumption. Attitudes to personality and adjustment often reflect negative images of increased and overwhelming introversion, of rigidity and 'bloody mindedness'. Again this common image is far from the reality.

The involvement of the clinical psychologist with intervention and treatment, support and guidance has actively increased with elderly groups as it has with other age groups. The techniques for handling, for example, normal adjustment problems, depression, anxiety and stress related difficulties and sexual disharmony, pioneered for use with a younger population, have been adapted for use with the elderly and found to be effective. Taken together these psychological approaches have much potential for adding to the quality of life for the elderly.

### Intellectual Functioning

Clinical psychologists have had a traditional role in the assessment of intellectual functioning and the interpretation of changes in aspects of this functioning. The effects of age on intellectual performance have been a matter for discussion since the earliest collections of 'behaviour samples' into intelligence tests. Whilst much earlier consideration concentrated on the developments of intellect in children the widespread use of intelligence tests in the First World War produced results which, for the first time, extended these discussions throughout the life-span.

The fifty-year period from 1916 to 1965 produced many studies on whole life intellectual development of which a typical summary would be that in the earlier editions of the classic textbook by Wechsler *The Measurement and Appraisal of Adult Intelligence.* A view of intellectual development emerged which placed strong emphasis on the apparent decline in abilities from a peak in the twenty to thirty age range. The 1972 edition of Wechsler's book (Matarazzo, 1972) suggests that this decline may be of the order of one-third of peak capacity.

This view of inevitable overall decline seems to accord with the expectancies of the man-in-the-street who has strong negative views of the elderly and an expectancy of intellectual decline. This inevitable decline model continues to be presented in texts for many professions including social work, nursing, and medicine.

The past fifteen years have seen a re-examination of these hypotheses. This has been assisted by an increasing awareness of the methodological factors influencing studies of age related change. This whole topic is too extensive to cover in detail here; the reader might consult a review such as appears in *The Handbook of the Psychology of Aging* (Botwinick, 1977). The main problem is that most of the traditional conclusions on decline were derived from cross-sectional studies which confound the age variable with other influences. Groups of different ages will have had different sociocultural backgrounds with a potential influence on their intellectual development. In the United Kingdom a useful illustrative variable is length of normal school education. This can vary with a school leaving age ranging from twelve to sixteen in today's population. Indeed our studies at Newcastle (Savage *et al.*, 1973) have shown that many of the older individuals were only intermittently in school after the age of ten.

Longitudinal studies, following the individual over a period of time are a possible alternative, although cultural changes may still prove something of a problem. These are particular difficulties when rapid changes, perhaps within a generation, affect the population studied. Longitudinal studies also raise practical problems such as continuity of finance and the danger that the tests or measures used may seem inappropriate to investigators in later years.

Various alternative models have been suggested which combine features of cross-sectional and longitudinal methodology. These enable inference to be made relating to age changes with a greater awareness of confounding issues, even if there is no 'perfect' experimental model. A few significant studies have emerged using either longitudinal or mixed models which have greatly influenced psychologists in the attitudes to intellectual changes with advancing age.

Schaie and Strother (1968) provided early evidence in a comparison of a cross-sectional and a mixed model which suggested strongly that overall decline was not a reasonable expectancy. The Newcastle-upon-Tyne group (Savage *et al.*, 1973) using simple longitudinal data did not find substantial decline in their studies. Recently results from a methodologically sophisticated study by Siegler and Botwinick (1979), which took features such as selective attrition of subjects into account, provided further evidence of a lack of overall decline in intellect. They say 'there is a sizeable proportion of old people who decline very little as old age advances or decline not at all, except perhaps in extreme old age'.

This would appear to be the current position and needs to be brought forcibly to the attention of those caring for the elderly. An expectation of decline as a matter of course in all old people is not justified by the evidence.

Two other features of interest relate to sub-groups within the aged population. The Newcastle studies suggest that there is an exceptionally well-preserved group of the aged, who seem to carry into old age their intellectual quality of life. There is also a suggestion that there may be a pre-death change in intellectual ability which is identifiable. The latter will be discussed later, the former is of interest in that this group could be used as a resource to provide care for their fellows.

**Personality and Adjustment**

Changes in personality with age have interested psychologists and their links with adjustment and life-satisfaction have been investigated. The 1960s saw a considerable interest in this topic and investigations attempting to produce models of age related change. Unfortunately, many of the methodological problems which we have considered in relation to changes in intellectual performance relate to this area as well. Similar difficulties occur in isolating age-related changes from cultural and environmental factors.

If one can produce a caricature of the personality and adjustment changes which our man-in-the-street expects in old age we find increased withdrawal, increased emotionality, anxiety, and other negatively evaluated features. This expectancy is likely to be general and cover all the aged.

The extensive review of personality and psychological adjustment studies of the 1960s and early 1970s carried out by Savage *et al.* (1977) suggests that the changes found tended to support the general picture above. Introversion appears to increase, anxiety and depressive behaviour likewise appear more frequently. However, the overwhelming characteristic of these studies is the variability of their findings. Compared with the intellectual behaviour there are far fewer clear-cut conclusions. It would appear that the research methodology has tended to obscure change and confuse interpretation.

Gaber (reported in Savage, 1977) evaluated a group of the aged on a variety of personality and life-satisfaction measures and produced interesting results. These were summarized in four basic groups.

Group I: Contained 54 per cent of the aged and were found to be comparable to younger groups in their personality. There were small and insignificant changes in introversion and anxiety, certainly no changes major enough seriously to affect adjustment.

Group II: Almost 20 per cent were noticeably more introverted and withdrawn.

Group III: Ten per cent of the sample were noticeably perturbed, suspicious, and emotionally unstable.

Group IV: Sixteen per cent of the sample were exceptionally well adjusted and reflected very little personality change.

This study is of interest in that it clearly suggests that it would be unreasonable to expect all the aged to reflect the negative changes in personality and adjustment which seem to be expected with advancing age. If we combine groups I and IV 70 per cent of the sample were well adjusted reflecting little personality change and reasonable life satisfaction. Again, as with some studies on intellectual change it is important to note the emergence of a noticeably well-preserved group of the aged.

The abnormal adjustment found in this study seems to separate into two distinct groups. The introverted tend to stick to themselves, retreat to their homes and internalize conflicts. They may well be a difficult group to identify as they will keep away from helping agencies. The perturbed, on the other hand, may well be constantly and actively seeking help, often to the stage of being over-demanding of relatives and care agencies.

Similar findings which appear in other recent studies confirm that it would be unfortunate to assume overall negative personality change with all old age. A substantial group of the aged show little personality change and adjust remarkably well to the demands of later life.

## Psychological Intervention

The past few years have seen a rapidly expanding interest in supporting the aged in their natural environment. Clinical psychologists can play a significant role in this exercise by applying their knowledge of the psychological changes to be expected and capitalizing on their increasing skills in behavioural intervention. The economics of the situation will increasingly dictate that expensive care of a whole-time nature be avoided if at all possible.

The changes in memory which may occur with ageing place increasing demands on the individual. Particular problems may be a reduction in memory capacity at input and recall. This area is readily open to prophylactic treatment based on our rapidly improving psychological knowledge of memory processes.

A good example is the potential for using cues to assist recall. The older person may well have markedly deficient free recall for important factors supporting day-to-day life, but be dramatically assisted by even the smallest cue. An illustration would be a cue board containing something like a daily timetable, for example:

| | |
|---|---|
| In the bedroom | — put on slippers |
| Wake up time | — put on dressing gown |
| | — go to kitchen |
| | — put on kettle |
| In the kitchen | — set out teapot, cup, etc. |
| Early morning | — put out pills |
| | etc., etc. |

Lists of this type, which can concentrate on the deficient areas, should be easily adaptable to individual circumstances, and are remarkably effective in assisting adjustment. The possibilities are wide and once the idea has been grasped the psychologist does not need intensive involvement, the family or often the client will build on the basic concept.

A recent client was helped in her baking by a simple ingredient cue list which reminded her of basic constituents. This seemingly small change encouraged her husband and herself to apply the same technique to other problem areas they both had, and a dramatic change in their personal relationship and general life satisfaction ensued.

At a more complicated level attempts have been made to apply microprocessors and microcomputers to these problems (Lyle, 1980). They can provide an interactive cue pattern with features such as relationship of cueing to time of the day built in. Thus many activities of daily living may be cued on a sophisticated alarm clock basis.

The vast range of behavioural techniques used in the community by psychologists are equally applicable to the aged. Among these are the techniques which assist independence and reduce stress. A wide range of problems can affect the elderly below the threshold of psychiatric referral and reduce the quality of life. There can be the pressing problems of anxiety or depression-related behaviour. Minor intervention can avoid this sort of problem developing into acute and disabling illness. All too often such features which would be identified and corrected in adulthood are ignored and untreated in the aged, leading to eventual maladjustment or even hospitalization.

Other areas of possible assistance include counselling and advice on family relationships and personal problems including sexual difficulties. Recent work by Stirling (1980) has suggested that many aspects of family therapy, developed in relation to children's problems, may be quite relevant to the family which incorporates an aged relative. All too often aged individuals are considered as separate units, and the overall dynamic of the family and environment ignored. A comprehensive approach can greatly assist positive adjustment.

Sexual difficulties and adjustment problems are by no means absent in the aged. Recent years have seen powerful techniques of marital and sexual therapy successfully applied to a wide range of adult problems. Only recently have active efforts been made to support the quality of marital and sexual functioning into old age. The psychological techniques are well established. Attitudinal change is more difficult, attempts to persuade doctors and care agents that sex after seventy is possible, fruitful and fulfilling, can at times verge on the hilarious.

An important factor in stable old age is the inevitable involvement with death, dying, and bereavement. This can rank alongside sex as a taboo topic in our society. Psychologists now are much more aware of the behavioural aspects of these topics and it is possible to facilitate adjustment by appropriate counselling. Bereavement counselling can greatly assist the return to positive adaptation by encouraging adaptive behaviour.

Pain is often a persistent feature of otherwise stable old age. Advances in pain control and an awareness of the psychological components is leading to increasing attempts to support those affected, particularly by chronic pain. This again is an area where techniques developed in relation to other age groups can be of obvious use to the aged.

This selection of possible areas for psychological intervention represents a few of the many possibilities. The main point to be emphasized is that it is essential to explore the possibility of using the whole range of psychological intervention and support techniques to assist the adjustment of the normal, stable aged person. In this way one can, hopefully maintain the quality of life for as long as possible. It is also necessary that these techniques are as widely publicized as possible so that the whole range of helping professions interacting with the aged are aware of their potential.

## PROBLEMS IN THE AGED

In the earlier sections we have explored aspects of stable old age and now must pass to a consideration of some of the specific problems and abnormal changes which may occur. These incorporate both qualitative and quantitative differences from stable ageing and pose specific problems for the caring professions and clinical psychology.

Traditionally, clinical psychology first encountered the aged in relation to these problems and abnormalities. Most large hospitals have their quota of wards full of demented, depressed, or otherwise highly problematical aged. The nature of these wards has been such as to deter even the most determined psychologist. However, in the 1960s the balance of care began to change with a considerable increase in local authority and NHS provision. This structured care was based on adequate assessment of both medical and behavioural difficulties.

The range of care available now varies from support in the home, through day hospitals, to sheltered housing. The elderly mentally infirm have their separate provision and the psychiatric hospital ward is very much a last resort. At all of these levels some psychologists have been playing an increasing part in assessment and care for many years. There is still a vast untapped area of greater psychologist involvement with much potential for an increase in the quality of life.

### Intellectual Deterioration

We have referred to the psychological finding that deterioration in intellectual processes is by no means a universal expectancy in the aged. However, in some individuals, deterioration does occur and has a marked influence on their lives. Deterioration may be the result of a wide range of processes, some general, some specific which affect brain function. A thorough review of this area is available in Miller's now classic book, *Abnormal Ageing: The Psychology of Senile and Presenile Dementia* (1977).

The nature and extent of intellectual change and its effect on behaviour have been extensively studied in recent times. Some of the findings are worthy of examination since they raise interesting possibilities. In an earlier part of this chapter when considering intellectual development we found that there was a small group of people with overt deterioration. The nature and extent of deterioration in this group of the aged has proved a useful area of study.

## The Concept of Terminal Decline

When the aged with overt intellectual deterioration are examined (Kay *et al.*, 1977) it is evident that they have a markedly reduced life expectancy. This raises the possibility of some process related to terminal decline, an idea which first appeared in the early 1960s. Our Newcastle studies on intellectual change (Savage *et al.*, 1973) examined this suggestion by following our aged group through to death. We then used time of death as the baseline and analysed our data with assessments arranged in months before deaths.

An interesting picture emerged of marked pre-death deterioration in intellectual processes with both the experiential, long-term, aspects of intellectual functioning and the immediate adaptive behaviour aspects deteriorating. This is a significant finding. Its practical implications are wide ranging, and include possible prediction of a terminal state. These findings related closely to the experiences of care agents which suggest that the normally accessible and stable aspects of intellect such as vocabulary and long term-memory deteriorate markedly before death. It would appear that when an old person *stops* being able to reminisce is the time to get really worried about survival.

Support for these findings has come from American studies by Botwinick *et al*. (1978). They reviewed the area finding evidence supporting the concept of terminal decline and conducted a study which found that a group of some thirteen psychological tests could predict early death. Important predictors included such items as maze tracing, digit-symbol substitution and vigilance tests, as well as self-ratings of health and depression rating scales. This concept of detection of terminal decline with psychological tests remains an active research issue. Should further studies produce stable evidence of patterns of change we will be faced with interesting practical and ethical issues in the application of the findings.

## Intellectual and Behavioural Assessment

The search for appropriate tests to distinguish aspects of intellectual change which are predictive has led from general intelligence measures to very specific tests derived from Experimental Psychology. Deterioration may manifest as a global problem but there is likely to be more benefit in distinguishing differential changes in long-term experiential abilities from changes in immediate adaptive abilities. Unfortunately, the psychological tests available in the early 1970s were not at all optimal as discriminators of specific psychological processes. Such discrimination is essential for directed treatment.

The past few years have seen a renewed interest in the construction of more appropriate psychological tests for the aged. These have drawn on vastly increased knowledge in such areas as information processing and neuropsychology. The availability of microcomputers to store, present, and analyse test material is a possibility currently being actively explored in many research units. This coming together of sound psychological theory and technology of presentation is likely to have much to offer for the future.

Two important new batteries of psychological tests for the aged have emerged in the United Kingdom in the past few years. They both attempt to assist in the identification and monitoring of change and are likely to have extensive practical application. They are the Kendrick Battery for the Detection of Dementia (Gibson and Kendrick, 1979) and the Clifton Assessment Procedures for the Elderly (Pattie and Gilliard, 1979).

The Kendrick Battery incorporates tests said to be those 'most sensitive to age changes; immediate recall of briefly perceived data; and speed processing and recording information'. The Clifton Procedures assess the client's current grasp of the intellectual process such as information/orientation and have further sections assessing adaptive behaviour and dependency. It is likely that specific scales such as these will have an increasing use in the future in the hands not only of psychologists but of a wide variety of care agents to assess and monitor change.

The concept of measurement of adaptive behaviour, exemplified in the Adaptive Behaviour Scales (Nihira, 1969), developed for use with the mentally handicapped has a considerable potential in the care of the elderly.

Once deterioration has occurred and dependency builds up one of the most important facets of assessment is the degree of independent functioning which remains for the individual. Assessment of remaining abilities in this area can be of crucial relevance to practical care and placement.

As yet there is no global scale which has been specifically devised for the elderly and widely accepted. However, there are many prototype scales of which an adaptation of the Crichton Geriatric Rating Scale by Woods (1979) is typical. It covers competence in these areas:

1. Orientation
2. Mobility
3. Feeding
4. Dressing
5. Continence
6. Interest in environment
7. Interest in others
8. Social behaviour
9. Restlessness
10. Co-operation
11. Sleep
12. Communication
13. Complaints

Scales of this type are essential if one is to initiate and monitor attempts at behavioural intervention. It is likely that much effort will be expended to produce more effective scales in the coming years.

Psychological assessment appeared to suffer a decline in the 1970s with attacks on the concept of intelligence and intelligence tests which had changed little since 1930. The 1980s are seeing a new assessment concept. This is closely related to the planning and monitoring of effective intervention and is founded on the vast knowledge of behaviour possessed by contemporary psychology integrated with new assessment technology.

**Aspects of Treatment**

Active psychological treatment of the behavioural problems encountered in abnormal ageing has increased markedly in the past few years. Some general journal articles in the late 1970s (Miller, 1977; Woods and Britton, 1977) reflected growing interest, as did a significant and substantive review article by Patterson and Jackson (1980). This article illustrated progress in the application of behavioural techniques across a broad range of difficulties encountered by the aged and evaluated the use of a wide variety of procedures.

Intervention and treatment with the aged necessarily involves the same problems as exist with any population. For example, facile attempts to induce behaviour change in alien environments, such as day centres, are likely to face identical problems of generalization and maintenance to those evident in younger people when the client returns home. Similarly, the attitudes of family, nurses, and other care staff must be taken into consideration and their ability to facilitate or destroy any programme evaluated. The efficacy of intellectual processes must be taken into account; it is unlikely that the client will be able to learn as quickly, or be quite as compliant as when younger.

Many attempts at improving the quality of life of elderly clients have been based on an assumption that care environments, sensory deficits, or ongoing dementing processes may result in some form of sensory deprivation which leads to maladjustment. The answer to these problems is seen in stimulation and activity programmes or attempts actively to promote engagement. Sensory stimulation programmes seem to produce some stabilization and may halt decline in institutionalized clients. However, it has been suggested that there are considerable difficulties in pursuing these or any types of treatment without specific psychological models which take into account the psychological context of the elderly.

This problem is illustrated by a study of Simpson *ét al.* (1981) which examined the relationship between engagement and depression in a residential home for the elderly. Depression is a significant problem in the elderly in both community and residential settings. It might be expected that an absence of stimulation related to overt disengagement from the activities of the home might be closely related to depressive symptomatology. The study did not find any link between overt disengagement and depression.

A more detailed examination of their conclusions suggests that there may be much to gain from considering covert as well as overt behaviour. The authors state 'the quiet individual who is apparently staring into space . . . may report recall of happy memories . . . which . . . may have considerable functional importance'. This suggests that the techniques of cognitive therapy may be as important with the elderly as they are with younger people. Cognitive therapy stresses the integration of modification of overt behaviours with modification of underlying thoughts or cognitions. As yet there has been very little direct application of such approaches to the treatment of the aged.

A psychological treatment approach which has dramatically caught the attention of those involved with the aged in the UK is Reality Orientation (RO). The past five years have seen many hospital and residential settings using RO programmes and attempting to evaluate them. RO is based on a rationale outlined by Folsom (1968) and is essentially an active attempt to re-orientate clients to their current environment. The programme may continue throughout the whole day or may be 'classroom based' in specific sessions. The client is continually reminded of orientation to day, time, and place; identity is reinforced and the environment external to the unit is emphasized (it is raining, look at the daffodils outside).

The full implementation of RO implies a massive change in ward or unit environment and uses considerable staff resources. Yet the procedures only deal with part of total adjustment, the area of orientation. Attempts to evaluate RO face the considerable difficulties which await those attempting to evaluate any behavioural treatment regime. Recent controlled studies (Woods, 1979; Hanley *et al.*, 1981) in the UK seem to suggest that RO may reduce deterioration in confused patients, but at the cost of massive resource input. It would seem that those who regard RO as the cornerstone of a treatment revolution for the confused elderly are perhaps a trifle premature. The real need is for some better theoretical rationale for intervention of this type.

In addition to specific techniques developed for the elderly a wide range of standard behaviour modification techniques have been applied to the elderly. Phobic symptoms can effect the aged and be as crippling as with younger patients. The effective techniques devised and proven with younger patients have been used with considerable success. Attempts to re-establish basic skills such as toilet training can be successful even in extreme old age and after considerable brain damage. Social skills and communication can be re-established. There is not scope in this chapter to add to these illustrations with detailed discussion and evidence. Examples have been given and the very firm point made that behavioural problems and disorders in the elderly can and must be approached with the same positive attitude, skills, and techniques as would be used with younger clients.

## OVERVIEW AND PROSPECT

Those topics which have been considered should indicate that clients covered by the narrow concept of 'psychogeriatrics' are among those who can be greatly assisted by the application of the clinical psychologist of his knowledge and skills. However, there is much more to be gained from a more general application of psychological techniques and awareness to a wider range of possibilities from retirement throughout all aspects of care of the aged.

It has been shown that retirement is not the simple concept it might have been a few years ago. Economic change has produced a life event which may occur from middle age onwards and which must be positively approached to obtain optimal adjustment for the future. Stable old age is *not* a time of inevitable intellectual deterioration and personality disintegration with little life satisfaction. On the contrary, most individuals can expect a fruitful period of years building on the foundation of adulthood.

Real problems do exist, mental illness can attack the aged, behavioural disorders may occur, dementia and strokes may intervene. However, as we become more aware of the psychological processes involved we are devising ever more potent treatment techniques which prolong the quality of life for as long as possible. Psychologists in the UK have been and will continue to be active in such development and as active in making others aware of the potential contribution of psychological knowledge to their own interactions with the aged.

## REFERENCES


Botwinick, J. (1977). Intellectual abilities. In J. E. Birren and K. W. Schaie (eds) *Handbook of the Psychology of Aging.* New York: Van Nostrand Reinhold.

Botwinick, J., West, R., and Storandt, M. (1978). Predicting death from behavioural test performance. *Journal of Gerontology,* **33**, 755–762.

Council of Europe (1977). *Preparation for Retirement.* Council of Europe.

Folsom, J. C. (1968). Reality orientation for the elderly mental patient. *Journal of Geriatric Psychiatry,* **1**, 291–307.

Gibson, A. J., and Kendrick, D. C. (1979). *The Kendrick Battery for the Detection of Dementia in the Elderly.* Windsor: NFER Publishing Co.

Hanley, I. G., McGuire, R. J., and Boy, O. W. D. (1981). Reality orientation and dementia: A controlled trial of two approaches. *British Journal of Psychiatry*, **138**, 10–14.

Kay, D. W. K., Britton, P. G., Bergmann, K., and Forster, M. (1977). Cognitive functioning and length of survival in elderly subjects living at home. *Australian and New Zealand Journal of Psychiatry,* **11**, 113–117.

Liddell, A., and Boyle, M. (1980). Characteristics of applicants to the M.Sc. in Clinical Psychology at NELP. *Newsletter of the Clinical Division of the British Psychological Society, No. 30*, 20–25.

Lyle, R. (1980). Prospect for an applied psychology for the elderly. *Proceedings of the Annual Conference of the British Psychological Society,* Aberdeen.

Matarazzo, J. D. (1972). *Wechsler's Measurement and Appraisal of Adult Intelligence*, 5th ed. Baltimore: Williams and Wilkins.

Miller, E. (1977). The management of dementia: A review of some possibilities. *British Journal of Social and Clinical Psychology,* **16**, 77–83.

Miller, E. (1977). *Abnormal Ageing: The Psychology of Senile and Presenile Dementia.* Chichester: Wiley.

Nihira, K. (1969). *The Adaptive Behavior Scales.* The American Association for Mental Deficiency.

Patterson, R. L., and Jackson, G. M. (1980). Behaviour modification with the elderly. *Progress in Behaviour Modification,* **9**, 205–239.

Pattie, A. H., and Gilliard, C. J. (1979). *The Clifton Assessment Procedures for the elderly.* Sevenoaks: Hodder and Stoughton.
Savage, R. D., Britton, P. G., Bolton, N., and Hall, E. H. (1973). *Intellectual Functioning of the Aged.* London: Methuen.
Savage, R. D., Gaber, L. B., Britton, P. G., Bolton, N., and Cooper, A. (1977). *Personality and Adjustment in the Aged*. London: Academic Press.
Schaie, K. W., and Strother, C. R. (1968). A cross-sequential study of age changes in cognitive behaviour. *Psychological Bulletin,* **70**, 671–680.
Schaie, K. W. (1965). A general model for the study of developmental problems. *Psychological Bulletin,* **64**, 92–107.
Siegler, K., and Botwinick, J. (1979). A long-term study of intellectual abilities of older adults — the matter of selective subject attrition. *Journal of Gerontology,* **34**, 242–247.
Simpson, S., Woods, R. T., and Britton, P. G. (1981). Depression and engagement in a residential home for the elderly. *Behaviour Research and Therapy,* **19**, 435–438.
Stirling, E. (1980). Tolerance of debility in elderly and chronically ill dependants by families in the community. Proceedings of the December Conference of the British Psychological Society. *Bulletin of The British Psychological Society,* **34**, 34.
Welford, A. T. (1951). *Skill and Age.* London: Oxford University Press.
Welford, A. T. (1958). *Ageing and Human Skill.* London: Oxford University Press.
Woods, R. T. (1979). Reality orientation and staff attention — controlled study. *British Journal of Psychiatry,* **134**, 502–507.
Woods, R. T., and Britton, P. G. (1977). Psychological approaches to the treatment of the elderly. *Age and Ageing,* **6**, 104–111.

The Practice of Clinical Psychology in Great Britain
Edited by A. Liddell


# *Chapter 12*

# *Physical handicap*

*Nadina Lincoln*

Although the number of clinical psychologists working with the physically handicapped is small there has already been diversification of the settings where they work and the role that they take. Initially they were almost exclusively based in specialist rehabilitation units and providing a service only for that unit. Now they provide an area based service covering young disabled units, homes for the disabled, special care units, and general hospital rehabilitation departments. Their role has also changed. The increasing tendency is for clinical psychologists to train other professions, such as physiotherapists and occupational therapists, in techniques of assessment and treatment, rather than work directly with patients.

The importance of psychological factors in physical handicap has long been recognized and motivation, personality, and attitudes are important determinants of whether a person adapts to his disability. These factors are being systematically investigated so that appropriate assessment and training techniques may be developed. The role of the psychologist has been to determine which variables affect the process of adaptation to disability and to determine how adaptation may be improved. They then train others in the use of these techniques, so that they may be applied to a larger proportion of patients.

The role of the clinical psychologist working with the physically handicapped will be considered under the following five headings:

1. Monitoring the effects of disability
2. General patient management
3. Specific training programmes
4. Evaluation of rehabilitation techniques
5. Adjustment to disability

## MONITORING THE EFFECTS OF DISABILITY

### Measurement of Disability and Handicap

There is increasing emphasis on the objective evaluation of the extent of physical disability and its associated handicap. This is needed in order to provide a basis for the allocation of services, to record progress, and to predict the outcome of rehabilitation. Because of their experience in the design of assessment techniques, clinical psychologists have become involved in the development of measurement techniques for other professions.

Two types of assessment are needed. One is the measurement of physical disability, that is the loss of function resulting from the medical condition. Examples are techniques to assess hand function (Lyle *et al.*, 1979), motor function in stroke patients (Lincoln and Leadbitter, 1979), and driving skills (Smith and Wilson, 1980).

The second type of assessment measures handicap, the social disadvantage which may result from the physical disability. For example, questionnaires have been designed to investigate the effects of memory impairment in head injury patients (Sunderland and Harris, 1980) and the effects of brain damage on personal and social life (Oddy *et al.*, 1978; Coughlan and Humphrey, 1980).

In addition, many of the assessments currently used by physiotherapists and occupational therapists are being improved by standardization of administration and scoring, such that a more objective interpretation of results may be possible. Hitherto, there has rarely been any evaluation of reliability of these measures, despite the fact that they are used by several different therapists and as measures of change. Clinical psychologists are helping to assess the reliability and validity of some of these assessments and thereby to create improved means of monitoring changes in ability, including the response to treatment.

## Psychological Assessments

Psychological assessments of a more traditional type are also carried out. These are generally to answer one of three questions:

1. What is this person's level of functioning, such that appropriate guidance may be given in relation to education or employment?
2. What cognitive abilities and disabilities does this person have which may affect his rehabilitation or require specific intervention?
3. Are there psychological factors associated with the physical disability which may affect this person's response to treatment or adaptation to disability?

The assessment of overall level of functioning in relation to education or employment is generally based on the standardized test procedures used with the non-physically disabled population, for example Wechsler Adult Intelligence Scale (Wechsler, 1955), and Progressive Matrices and Mill Hill Vocabulary (Raven, 1958). Allowances are made according to the type of disability but these are rarely standardized and normative data are not usually available for the modified versions of the tests. Such data need to be collected if standard tests are to be widely used with a physically disabled population. However, the advantage of the present system is that it shows how a disabled person will compare with the general population if no allowances can be made for his disability.

Assessments of cognitive abilities and disabilities suffer less from the limitation imposed by physical disability because there is a wider variety of tests available covering the major cognitive categories. If the patient has motor speech difficulties verbal abilities may be assessed on written tasks such as the Mill Hill Vocabulary (Raven, 1958). If he is unable to write, the synonyms section of this can sometimes be carried out using a pointer. Although written forms of the comprehension and similarities tests of the WAIS may not be exactly equivalent to the spoken version, they usually provide sufficient information for the referral question to be answered. Ideally, appropriate normative data should be obtained. Visuospatial abilities are usually assessed on the Block Design of the WAIS or copying the Rey–Osterreith figure (Rey, 1959). However, if the patient has insufficient manual dexterity for these tasks, there are other tests available, include Cube Counting (Ratcliff, 1970), Incomplete Pictures (Gollin, 1960), and Unusual Views (Warrington, unpublished). Memory testing presents further problems. Writing answers to verbal memory tasks such as the Wechsler Logical Memory (Wechsler and Stone, 1945) is rarely used because the time from hearing to recall is longer than in oral tests. Other tests of verbal memory which are more often used are Williams Delayed Recall (Williams, 1968) and the Forced Choice Words Test (Warrington, 1974). Visual memory tests usually involve drawing geometric forms, but there are alternatives such as the multiple choice version of the Benton Visual Retention Test (Benton, 1950), Warrington non-verbal retention test (Warrington and James, 1967), and a Forced Choice Faces Recognition. Some patients, particularly those with multiple sclerosis, also have poor visual acuity, which makes these tasks impossible. For this reason Staples and Lincoln (1981) devised a maze learning test, requiring only sufficient vision to see whether a light was on and sufficient motor control to operate a lever, to test visual memory.

Although the modifications in test procedure needed are likely to have some effect on test scores, it is usually possible to get sufficient information to be able to answer the referral question in general terms. The broad areas of difficulty may be identified but the precision and analysis of deficits used for neuropsychological investigation of patients is not generally possible in the presence of severe physical handicap.

Investigation of psychological factors associated with physical disability has been extensive but has yielded relatively little of direct clinical relevance. Studies have attempted to identify psychological concomitants of disabilities. Thus, there have been attempts to identify a particular personality profile associated with a disability, such as rheumatoid arthritis or asthma. It has been suggested that these abnormal personality profiles may in some way predispose the person to a particular disease. However, the studies are generally inconclusive (Shontz, 1971) and the information gathered has not generally proved clinically useful. The one clinical situation where personality tests are occasionally used is in an attempt to differentiate organic from functional disorders, particularly in chronic low back pain patients. However, although several studies have been conducted on personality features of low back pain patients (Grzesiak, 1980), they have failed to provide an adequate means of distinguishing those with organic pathology from those without. Most psychologists use the Eysenck Personality Inventory and rating scales such as the Zung Self-rating Depression Scale (Zung, 1965), Middlesex Hospital Questionnaire (Crown and Crisp, 1970), and Goldberg General Health Questionnaire (Goldberg, 1972), in an attempt to answer the question rather than the MMPI, which was used for most experimental studies. One centre is using the Eysenck Personality Questionnaire for patients attending a spinal disorders clinic in an attempt to improve the diagnosis of patients with psychogenic problems presenting as back pain (Seal, 1979).

The other purpose of psychological assessments with patients in various disability groups has been to identify those likely to make a poor response to rehabilitation. If such people can be identified it may be possible to alter the rehabilitation programme in accordance with their difficulty. Measures of attitudes, beliefs, and mood tend to be used in this situation rather than measures of personality. In a study of patients with rheumatoid arthritis Gardiner (1980) found that those who rated themselves as 'slow, dependent, and weak' lost more time off work in the subsequent year. Since attitudes were not found to be related to the physical progression of the disease, it would suggest that such psychological variables affect the outcome of rehabilitation. Similar results were obtained with a group of chronic bronchitics (Rutter, 1976). In this study scores on the Zung Self-rating Depression Scale (Zung, 1965) were significantly related to unemployment and poor work record whereas independent objective assessment of physical disability did not.

Another predictive variable to have been considered includes one aspect of a person's beliefs about himself, his locus of control. Brewin and Shapiro (1979) suggest that patients with an external locus of control are less likely to respond to rehabilitation than those with an internal locus of control. The implications of this suggestion were that therapists and patients should agree goals and targets which may be readily understood by the patient and let him feel that he is making progress in an objective quantifiable way. It is argued that patients who are educated to make their own decisions about their goals and their future are more likely to develop a sense of personal control and ability to change. It, therefore, seems that the predictive value of the person's locus of control is very much dependent on the nature of the rehabilitation programme in which he is engaged.

Although such measures may suggest those who will respond poorly to rehabilitation they have not been tested sufficiently in clinical practice. The type of intervention and whether it has any effect on these likely poor responders has yet to be determined. Nevertheless these approaches seem to have more direct clinical application than the examination of personality profiles.

### Special Assessment Techniques

Some of the physically handicapped are too disabled for any of the assessment techniques mentioned so far to be appropriate. Those who have only very minimal movements, together with no speech, blindness, or deafness cannot be assessed on standard tasks. Special assessments have to be devised according to their disability and in general terms the questions to be answered are much more basic. For example: 'Can this person understand what is going on around him?', 'Can he learn to communicate in any way?', or 'What can he learn to do that will provide some sort of occupation or entertainment?'.

The first object is the provision of some means by which a response may be obtained. A variety of switches have been developed for disabled people to operate environmental controls or communication aids, such as a Possum typewriter. These switches can be adapted to operate other devices, such as lights, buzzers, and radios and to provide feedback of the response. Once some means of response has been established it is possible to test auditory and visual comprehension to some extent by providing instructions and a response code. For example, visual matching can be assessed using a response code such as 'one press for same, two for different'. Training may be necessary on very simple items before it is possible to assess more complex tasks. If the person does not have sufficient movement to operate a switch he may be trained using biofeedback techniques. For example, increase in EMG level may be obtainable when no recordable movement is present. Such recording techniques have wider application and can provide a means of communication or can be linked to environmental controls. For example, a head injury patient may be trained to respond using EMG biofeedback and once this is done, it is possible to assess hearing threshold and verbal comprehension of instructions, and it may then be possible to establish some means of communication. Similar devices for use in assessment and treatment are reviewed by Freidlander (1980).

Special assessment techniques are also needed for particular problems associated with disability. With technical advances, driving is becoming a practical possibility for more and more disabled people. However, although the technical problems can be solved, little account has been taken so far of the effect of acquired intellectual impairment on driving skills. If the disabled person has intellectual impairment as well as motor deficits these may present difficulties returning to driving. A preliminary investigation of stroke patients (Smith and Wilson, 1980) suggests that those who have returned to driving make more mistakes on a test track than age matched controls, and that they also perform worse on some tests of intellectual function. It is hoped that it will be possible to develop a screening assessment which will select patients with cognitive impairments likely to affect driving ability so that they may have adequate practical assessment and training before returning to drive.

### Future Developments

Current assessment techniques are mainly concerned with measuring the extent of physical disability. A problem which is beginning to be tackled is how to measure the effect which such disabilities have on people's lives. The handicap associated with a disability is probably a more useful evaluation of the effects of rehabilitation than the severity of the disability. However, even those disability measures which are available are rarely sufficiently standardized and reliable for our needs, and further work is being conducted on these.

The development of assessments is also being more oriented towards those with direct practical application. A measure of memory in multiple sclerosis patients which identifies those whose daily life is likely to be affected by the problem and for whom training is appropriate is more useful than one which is only an excellent discriminator between patients with multiple sclerosis and the general population.

Several attempts have been made to devise measures which predict response to rehabilitation. But this seems a little premature when we do not know what aspects of rehabilitation influence the course of recovery. If a particular measure predicted outcome in a particular group of patients, unless we know the effectiveness of the different component treatments, it is unlikely to be possible to use it as a predictor for another group of patients in a different hospital, with different therapists using different techniques. It is necessary first to establish what effect different treatment programmes have on promoting recovery or preventing deterioration. Predictive measures, while of interest, have not generally been applied by clinical psychologists.

## GENERAL PATIENT MANAGEMENT

One of the most frequent requests to a clinical psychologist working with the physically handicapped is to advise care staff on the management of patients. The problems presented include those of patients who have difficulties in accepting their disabilities, who are unco-operative with treatment, poorly motivated, unrealistic in their aims or aggressive and disruptive. These occur at any stage between the onset of the disability and the final discharge from hospital care, in long-stay residential accommodation or in the patient's own home. Whenever the problem is presented to the psychologist it is likely that patient management in the early stages of disability will have had an effect.

Therefore, much attention is being directed towards the management of recently disabled patients.

If the onset of a disability is sudden, it may be characterized by a period of confusion, disorganization, and aggression. Psychologists have sometimes adopted a crisis management policy of the type outlined by Fordyce (1971) to help the patient and his family through this phase. This consists of providing calm stable models for the patient and his family to emulate. Also, promoting performance mastery by providing carefully chosen tasks on which the patient can succeed. Patients may be aggressive, possibly because there are many punishment contingencies operating. Reinforcers which previously maintained their work and leisure activities are no longer available and instead they receive punishment, in the form of pain, physical discomfort or social disapproval, when trying to do new activities. By being aggressive, either physically or verbally, towards therapists the patient may escape from a situation which draws attention to his disability. If this is the case attempts are made to ignore the aggressive behaviour and at the same time using shaping procedures to increase participation in rehabilitation.

In addition psychologists are attempting to draw attention to other relevant aspects of acute care outlined by Michael (1970). He points out that attention and sympathy are contingent on behaviour, generally verbal, which indicates discontent, pain, and sadness. Attention is less often directed towards those who appear contented and happy, and who are quiet. The patient — staff ratio is usually such that attention is given to those in trouble or who request care, whereas those who are coping are ignored.

Another problem outlined by Fordyce is the tendency for carers to encourage the patients to adopt a role of unquestioning obedience; being told what to do and when. In this way a pattern of strong dependency is rewarded. Since these tendencies often cannot be changed on an acute hospital ward, it is important that if they do occur they are identified and reversed as early as possible.

Once the patient has begun on a rehabilitation programme the most likely problem which may be encountered is one of poor motivation. These patients do not do as much as they are expected to do, or do not progress as well as is expected. They may also refuse to co-operate with treatment. Much of the therapist's time is spent in coping with the patient rather than using her own specialist treatment skills. Therefore, programmes are set up based on target setting with attention, rest and feedback of progress contingent on successful completion of target behaviours. There are several examples of this type of general management approach in the literature (Goodkin, 1966; Michael, 1970; Ince, 1976).

General management problems may also occur in residential settings, including the patient's own home. This may reflect a failure of rehabilitation to transfer a patient from a dependent to an independent role, a transfer which should be attempted even in those with severe physical dependence. Patients who need long-term physical care over a period of many years may have been forced into a dependent role for so many daily activities, that they cease to be as independent as they could be.

Initial work with relatives or carers may involve encouragement of patients to make progressively more of their own decisions. For example, in the early stages this may include deciding what to wear, where in the room to sit and what to eat, even though they cannot physically manage to do these things themselves.

## SPECIFIC TRAINING PROGRAMMES

Specific programmes are set up to deal with individual rehabilitation problems. There are four main types:

1. Behaviour modification
2. Skills training
3. Cognitive retraining
4. Biofeedback

### Behaviour Modification

If the general management principles described in the previous section are insufficient to overcome a particular behaviour problem then a specific behaviour modification programme may be set up. If progress is slow patients may become discouraged or feel that the activities they are required to do will not meet their own aims. For example, a woodworking apprentice attending a rehabilitation workshop following a head injury became uncooperative and aggressive during woodwork sessions. He became unco-operative because he considered the tasks he was being given to do were too easy, whereas the occupational therapists considered him unfit to return to work because he was slow and inaccurate. A programme was designed to increase both his work speed and accuracy. A graded series of targets were devised which involved spending progressively longer on a routine woodwork task, making boxes. In addition the number of stages to be completed within the allotted time was increased. Points were awarded for the amount of work completed in the time limit, and deductions were made for specific inaccuracies, for example nail bent, corners not square. Points were exchanged for various leisure activities, and in addition a graph kept of his progress to provide additional reinforcement. His work speed increased from making one box in two half-hour sessions to eight boxes in one two-hour session. Initially, 100 per cent of points earned had to be deducted, but after the six week treatment period no deductions were necessary. Many examples of this type are quoted by Michael (1970), Ince (1976, 1980), and Fordyce (1976).

Generally psychologists using this approach have not carried out evaluations in comparison with other treatment methods. They have mainly been concerned with gaining experience in the application of behaviour modification in rehabilitation, and at best only using AB designs to evaluate the effects. Behaviour modification is becoming widely used in physical rehabilitation and further evaluation of its contribution is needed.

One major rehabilitation problem for which behaviour modification is used is in the management of chronic low back pain. Fordyce (1976) describes in detail a programme for patients with chronic low back pain with no or insufficient physical damage to account for its severity or persistence. It is based on the idea that pain behaviours may be reinforced by their consequences and over a prolonged period a whole repertoire of learned pain behaviours, including the subjective experience of pain, may be established. In other words, the patient may learn that a complaint of pain or disability leads to sympathy and help, whereas failure to complain does not. The programme aims to reverse this process by non-reinforcement of pain behaviours and reinforcement of activity. In addition, analgesics are given on a time-contingent rather than a pain-contingent basis. Results obtained by Fordyce (1976) indicate that pain behaviours may be reduced and activity increased, although in this instance no record was made of the effect of the programme on subjective pain. A pilot study by Silverman (1976) suggested that subjective pain either remained constant or improved, even though patients were doing more. Programmes of this type are being used in rehabilitation centres for low back pain and have been found to be useful. The continuous monitoring of progress means that patients may be treated on condition that they continue to improve and discharged once improvement ceases. In a group, characterized by repeatedly failing treatment and being passed from one specialist to another, this ensures that therapist time is only being spent if some gains are being made. Whether the apparently good response is due to the actual treatment policy or whether it is just due to the patients being treated by someone who feels they may benefit, remains to be determined. However, chronic low back pain patients have long been a major rehabilitation problem and represent a large proportion of disabled patients so that any advance in their treatment is of significant practical benefit.

## Skills Training

A large proportion of time during the rehabilitation stage involves teaching patients to perform familiar skills in different ways, such as dressing for a hemiplegic patient, or learning new skills such as propelling a wheelchair or walking with an artificial leg. Most patients acquire these skills with practice, but if problems arise the clinical psychologist may be asked to advise on teaching methods. One of the most common reasons for failure to acquire the skill is that the patient has impaired learning ability as well as a physical disability. The task of the psychologist is to break down the skill into simple stages, with progress to the next stage dependent on successful acquisition of the previous stage. Frequent successes are ensured by keeping the stages simple and numerous. For example, in training wheelchair control the stages might be to propel a chair increasing distance in a given length of time. The difficulty of the task may be increased by restricting the available width of the route and presenting obstacles to be avoided. A similar approach may be used to train an elderly amputee to walk with an artificial leg or a stroke patient with visuospatial problems to dress.

## Cognitive Retraining

Many physical handicaps have associated intellectual deficits, for example memory and reasoning difficulties in multiple sclerosis, visuospatial problems with cerebral palsy, language or perceptual problems with strokes. These cognitive deficits may be amenable to retraining. Two main approaches are used; one is to attempt to train the area of deficit, for example, by practice on perceptual spatial tasks; the other is to train the patient to circumvent the problems associated with a particular deficit, for example, training patients to use verbal instructions rather than spatial abilities, to find their way around. Which of the two is used depends to some extent on the severity of the deficit, though they can be used in conjunction with each other.

The three cognitive areas for which treatments have been developed for deficits are in language, visuospatial abilities, and memory, though others such as reasoning and sequencing have been considered. Language treatments have until recently been exclusively carried out by speech therapists, but the development of programmed instruction and verbal conditioning procedures for aphasics had led to some collaboration between psychologists and speech therapists. The efficacy of either approach with aphasic patients remains doubtful (Sarno *et al.,* 1970; Lincoln *et al.*, 1982) and this has led to the development of new treatment approaches. Visual communication using symbols or sign language has been attempted, and though the gains made are small they may be greater than those achieved by conventional methods. Melodic Intonation Therapy (Albert *et al.*, 1973) and Brain Function Therapy (Buffery, 1977) are both based on the idea of stimulating the right hemisphere to take over language functions from the damaged left hemisphere. These have both been found useful with single cases but there seem to have been no investigations of their effectiveness compared with alternative treatment methods.

Perceptual training is a more recent development than that of language rehabilitation and most of that done by psychologists is based on the work of Diller and his colleagues (Diller, 1971, 1980). Defective visual scanning was selected for treatment. The initial aim was to make the patients aware of the difficulty and then to teach them to scan using an external stimulus which was sufficiently attractive to force the patients to turn their heads to the affected side. Diller developed a scanning machine, which requires the patient to point to a moving target. The patient has to learn to move his head when stimuli move to the left so that they come within the right visual field. Comparison of this procedure with conventional occupational therapy training indicated a beneficial effect, particularly in those with the most severe problems. Following training in scanning, treatments for spatial and sensory awareness were introduced with some patients. These consisted of matching a point touched on the patient's back with that on a manikin placed in front of the patient, and practice in estimating distances in space. Again, it was found that the treated group performed better than controls after one month's training.

Some psychologists are attempting to use these techniques with stroke and head injury patients but it is too early to judge their usefulness or effectiveness. However, it seems an area likely to develop because perceptual problems are common among stroke patients and yet are rarely identified or treated. The question yet to be answered is whether improvement acquired from training on these types of tasks is carried into performance in day-to-day living. It may be more appropriate to attempt retraining in real life situations, or it may be that both approaches should be used to help the patient to overcome the practical difficulties associated with perceptual–spatial problems.

Two different approaches are also used in memory training. In one patients are trained in strategies to aid memory using, for example, visual imagery and mnemonic aids. Thus, Wilson (1980) attempted to train a man with memory problems, which followed a head injury, to remember the names of the staff in the rehabilitation unit using visual imagery, to remember a shopping list using an initial letter mnemonic, and to remember routes between different places using verbal cueing. The visual imagery and initial letter mnemonic produced improvements in the patient's performance, whereas the verbal cueing did not.

The alternative approach, which tends to be used with those who have more severe memory loss, is to train them to circumvent the problem. In the initial stages patients are required to tick off the days of the week and particular times of day on a wall chart. This chart thus provides a reference to enable them to find out the day and time. Later, this is extended to the form of a daily diary, where events, such as activities completed in physiotherapy and occupational therapy and meals, are recorded at regular intervals throughout the day. Patients are encouraged to refer to their diary when discussing events that have happened and when planning treatment with their therapist. The planning of future events can then be incorporated into the diary. Each week the patient plans out a daily timetable in detail and is required to follow this timetable instead of asking what to do and where to go. Some patients with writing problems cannot cope with recording the information themselves, but they can be trained to refer to wall charts specifying what they should be doing and when. The benefits of this approach are that it can be easily adapted to everyday situations and is acceptable to relatives who find providing constant reminders very tedious.

Reality orientation training may also be appropriate for those with memory loss. Although mostly used with elderly demented patients, it may also be appropriate for those with similar problems associated with physical handicaps. Young disabled units often have large numbers of patients with memory problems. Reality orientation training on a 24-hour basis together with specific techniques of visual imagery and mnemonic aids might be used to help ameliorate some of their difficulties.

**Biofeedback**

The main type of biofeedback that has been used with the physically handicapped is electromyographic feedback for neuromuscular re-education. There are single case reports of successful treatment of a variety of clinical problems, including upper motor neurone lesions, Bell's palsy, and poliomyelitis. Some studies have compared biofeedback with alternative treatments (Brucker, 1980). In addition, Burnside *et al.* (1979) evaluated EMG feedback in the treatment of chronic foot drop with 22 stroke patients who were residents in Social Services Old Peoples Homes. Subjects were given either twelve sessions of EMG feedback training or twelve sessions of muscle tension recording with no feedback, while all were given exercises to practise between sessions. The number of patients who improved in range of movement and gait were not significantly different between the groups at the end of treatment, although at six weeks follow-up the biofeedback group was significantly better. The strength ratings showed that appreciably more people in the biofeedback group improved and this was maintained at follow-up. This study suggests that EMG biofeedback is an appropriate treatment with stroke patients and gains can be made without a lengthy or elaborate treatment programme.

However, further evaluation is needed. It may be possible to make significant progress in training to alleviate foot drop thereby producing functional gain whereas training hand and arm function may require greater increase in strength before significant functional gain is obtained. In clinical practice biofeedback can be used to demonstrate improvement in EMG levels, but it only rarely produces an improvement in patients' personal independence. The question then arises whether biofeedback training is worthwhile in terms of the practical gains made, and further studies are needed on different disabilities and involving different groups of muscles. As a treatment technique for clinical psychologists biofeedback seems likely to be useful, but continuous monitoring of progress, using single case experimental designs, is essential.

## EVALUATION OF REHABILITATION TECHNIQUES

Most rehabilitation techniques have developed over many years with little or no evaluation of their effectiveness. Those which have been found clinically useful have survived, but the problem is that many disabled patients improve or deteriorate independently of any intervention. It is then difficult to assess what has produced the observed changes. Such studies which have been completed have frequently had methodological faults, for example the major studies to evaluate speech therapy with stroke patients (Sarno *et al.*, 1970; Basso *et al.*, 1979). The need for evaluation of treatment effectiveness has become increasingly recognized and psychologists have become involved in both study design and in the teaching of research methods. Control group studies usually involve specific research staff and although essential do not involve many remedial therapists. On the other hand the application of single case experimental designs is a more straightforward undertaking and can be incorporated into the treatment regimes of physiotherapists, occupational therapists, and speech therapists. This latter approach at least enables therapists to identify some of the essential components of rehabilitation. However, if psychologists are to do this, then they have to ensure that psychological techniques introduced into rehabilitation do not meet with the same criticisms as earlier studies.

## ADJUSTMENT TO DISABILITY

Once the rehabilitation phase is completed and the patient has achieved his maximum level of independence, the problems referred to the psychologist tend to be those of failure to adjust to life as a disabled person. In some cases this also involves the adjustment of the spouse or relative.

The types of problem encountered include social anxieties, marital disharmony, sexual problems, over-reliance on professional help, and negative attitudes towards the self as a disabled person. Many of the techniques used by psychologists in a psychiatric setting can be directly applied to aiding the disabled in their social adjustment. For example, systematic desensitization can be used to help overcome anxieties about going into public places in a wheelchair, cognitive therapy can be used to reduce negative thoughts about themselves and their disabilities, and behavioural contracting can be used for marital problems.

Group therapy, in various forms, is being used to deal with many adjustment problems. Some groups serve an educational function in order for disabled people to discuss practical problems and to share ways of solving them. Others include relatives and may have a social as well as educational function. The relatives of some disabled patients may suffer as much of the isolation and practical limitations on life as the disabled person himself. Support groups for relatives are frequently as important as those for the patients. All the groups aim to get members to rely as much on self-help as possible and to wean them, as far as is practical, from obtaining help from professional sources. The role of the psychologist in these instances has generally been to initiate the formation of the groups rather than having any direct therapeutic role within the group setting. However, since recent studies on the social and psychological consequences of brain damage (Oddy *et al.*, 1978; Coughlan and Humphrey, 1979; Kansella and Duffy, 1979) suggest that major adjustment problems do occur, a more direct therapeutic role may develop.

The one area where psychologists may take a specific therapeutic role with the long-term disabled person is by providing sexual counselling. Physical disability besides its physical effects on sexual functioning often has psychological effects as well. Disability may render a person sexually unattractive in his own or his partner's opinion. In these cases discussion of the feelings and reactions to the disability may be sufficient. In others a graded approach, similar to that outlined by Masters and Johnson (1970), can be used to overcome fears and concern about how the partners will cope. In disabilities such as stroke or head injury, there may be initial loss of sexual functioning with gradual recovery. If the couple are not aware of this, impotence in the early stages of recovery may discourage either partner from further attempts at intercourse or create anxieties which in turn result in a persistence of the problem due to psychological rather than physical causes. A psychological approach to counselling may produce improvement even though the original problem was purely physical.

## CONCLUSION

Clinical psychologists are involved increasingly in the management of the physically handicapped. They are involved more in primary patient care, based in the community or in residential centres, and there is room for their greater involvement in acute hospital wards and in general hospital rehabilitation units. While desirable, this wider practice should not be to the detriment of their work in specialized rehabilitation centres, for their main role is to train others in the use of psychological techniques.

One of the greatest contributions that will continue to be made by clinical psychologists is to emphasize to therapists who work with the physically handicapped, the need for accurate assessment of the value of treatment programmes, and to teach them how such assessments may be made. Thus, although not a large professional group, clinical psychologists have an important and developing role within the multidisciplinary rehabilitation team.

## REFERENCES

Albert, M. L., Sparks, R. W., and Helm, N. A. (1973). Melodic intonation therapy for aphasia. *Archives of Neurology,* **29**, 130–131.

Basso, A., Capitani, E., and Vignolo, L. A. (1979). The influence of rehabilitation on language skills in aphasic patients: A controlled study. *Archives of Neurology*, **36**, 190–196.

Benton, A. L. (1950). A multiple choice type of the visual retention test. *Archives of Neurology and Psychiatry,* **64**, 699–707.

Brewin, C. R. and Shapiro, D. A. (1979). Beliefs about the self and their importance for motivation in rehabilitation. In D. J. Osborne, M. M. Gruneberg and J. R. Eiser (eds), *Research in Psychology and Medicine, Vol. II.* London: Academic Press.

Brucker, B. (1980). Biofeedback and rehabilitation. In L. P. Ince (ed.), *Behavioral Psychology in Rehabilitation Medicine.* Baltimore: Williams and Wilkins.

Buffery, A. W. H. (1977). Clinical neuropsychology: A review and preview. In S. Rachman (ed.), *Contributions to Medical Psychology.* London: Pergamon Press.

Burnside, I. G., Tobias, H. S., and Bursill, D. (1979). Electromyographic feedback in the remobilisation of stroke patients. In D. J. Osborne, M. M. Gruneberg and J. R. Eiser (eds), *Research in Psychology and Medicine Vol II.* London: Academic Press.

Coughlan, T., and Humphrey, M. (1980). Psychosocial problems in the rehabilitation of stroke patients. Paper presented to the Society for Research in Rehabilitation, Exeter, 10–11 July.

Crown, S., and Crisp, A. H. (1970). *The Middlesex Hospital Questionnaire Manual.* Barnstable: Psychological Test Publications.

Diller, L. (1971). Cognitive and motor aspects of handicapping conditions in the neurologically impaired. In W. S. Neff (ed.), *Rehabilitation Psychology.* Washington, D. C.: APA.

Diller, L. (1980). The development of a perceptual-remediation program in hemiplegia. In L. P. Ince (ed.), *Behavioral Psychology in Rehabilitation Medicine.* Baltimore: Williams and Wilkins.

Fordyce, W. E. (1971). Psychological assessment and management. In F. M. Krusen, F. J. Kottke and P. M. Ellwood (eds), *Handbook of Physical Medicine and Rehabilitation.* New York: Saunders.

Fordyce, W. E. (1976). *Behavioral Methods for Chronic Pain and Illness.* St Louis: Mosby.

Freidlander, B. Z. (1980). Automated operant methods for assessment and treatment in physical rehabilitation. In L. P. Ince (ed.), *Behavioral Psychology in Rehabilitation Medicine: Clinical Application*. Baltimore: Williams and Wilkins.
Gardiner, B. M. (1980). Psychological aspects of rheumatoid arthritis. *Psychological Medicine*, **10**, 159–165.
Goldberg, D. P. (1972). *The Detection of Psychiatric Illness by Questionnaire*. Maudsley Monograph No. 21. London: Oxford University Press.
Gollin, E. S. (1960). Development studies of visual recognition of incomplete objects. *Perceptual and Motor Skills*, **11**, 289–298.
Goodkin, R. (1966). Case studies in behavioural research in rehabilitation. *Perceptual and Motor Skills*, **23**, 171–182.
Grzesiak, R. C. (1980). Chronic pain: A psychobehavioral perspective. In L. P. Ince (ed.), *Behavioral Psychology in Rehabilitation Medicine: Clinical Applications*. Baltimore: Williams and Wilkins.
Ince, L. P. (1976). *Behavior Modification in Rehabilitation Medicine*. C. C. Thomas: Springfield, Illinois.
Ince, L. P. (1980). *Behavior Psychology in Rehabilitation Medicine*. Baltimore: Williams and Wilkins.
Kansella, G. J. and Duffy, F. D. (1979). Psychosocial readjustment in the spouses of aphasic patients. *Scandinavian Journal of Rehabilitation Medicine*, **II**, 129–132.
Lincoln, N. B., and Leadbitter, D. (1979). Assessment of motor function in stroke patients. *Physiotherapy*, **65**, 48–51.
Lincoln, N. B., Pickersgill, M. J., Hankey, A. I., and Hilton, C. R. (1982). An evaluation of operant training and speech therapy in the language rehabilitation of moderate aphasics. *Behavioural Psychotherapy*, **10**, 162–178.
Lyle, R. C., Stone, J., Meill, D. and Stewart, M. (1979). Abbreviation of ADL Testing by Gutman Scaling Techniques. Paper presented at a scientific meeting of the Society for Research in Rehabilitation, Newcastle-upon-Tyne, July 1979.
Masters, W. H., and Johnson, V. E. (1970). *Human Sexual Inadequacy*. Boston: Little, Brown.
Michael, J. L. (1970). Rehabilitation. In C. Neuringer and J. Michael (eds), *Behavior Modification in Clinical Psychology*. New York: Appleton-Century-Crofts.
Oddy, M., Humphrey, M., and Uttley, D. (1978). Subjective impairment and social recovery after closed head injury. *Journal of Neurology, Neurosurgery and Psychiatry*, **41**, 611–616.
Ratcliff, G. (1970). Aspects of disordered space perception. Unpublished Doctoral thesis, University of Oxford.
Raven, J. C. (1958). *Standard Progressive Matrices and Mill Hill Vocabulary*. London: Lewis.
Rey, A. (1959). *Le Test de Copie de Figure Complexe*. Paris: Editions centre de psychologie appliquee.
Rutter, B. M. (1976). Measurement of psychological factors in chronic illness. *Rheumatology and Rehabilitation*, **15**, 174–178.
Sarno, M. T., Silverman, J., and Sands, E. (1970). Speech therapy and language recovery in severe aphasia. *Journal of Speech and Hearing Research*, **13**, 607–623.
Seal, P. V. (1979). Early impressions from the use of the Eysenck Personality Questionnaire in patients attending a spinal disorders clinic. Lecture to the Society for Back Pain Research, London.
Shontz, F. C. (1971). Physical disability and personality. In W. S. Neff (ed.), *Rehabilitation Psychology*. Washington D.C.: APA.
Silverman, L. (1976). Behavioural management of chronic low back pain. Paper presented at course on low back pain, Rivermead Rehabilitation Centre, Oxford.
Smith, T., and Wilson, B. (1980). Personal Communication.
Staples, D., and Lincoln, N. B. (1981). A Maze Learning Test of Memory for the use

with Disabled Patients. Submitted for publication.

Sunderland, A., and Harris, J. (1980). Personal Communication.

Warrington, E. K. (1974). Deficient recognition in organic amnesia. *Cortex,* **10**, 289–291.

Warrington, E. K., and James, M. (1967). Disorders of visual perception in patients with localised lesions. *Neuropsychologia,* **5**, 253–366.

Wechsler, D. (1955). *Wechsler Adult Intelligence Scale.* New York: Psychological Corporation.

Wechsler, D., and Stone, C. (1945). *Wechsler Memory Scale.* New York: Psychological Corporation.

Williams, M. (1968). The measurement of memory in clinical practice. *British Journal of Social and Clinical Psychology,* **7**, 19–34.

Wilson, B. (1980). A single case experiment on memory training. Lecture given at a course on Research Methods for the Remedial Professions, Mary Marlborough Lodge, Oxford, November 19–20.

Zung, W. W. K. (1965). A self-rating depression scale. *Archives of General Psychiatry,* **12**, 63–70.

The Practice of Clinical Psychology in Great Britain
Edited by A. Liddell


## *Chapter 13*

# *Primary health care*

*Andrée Liddell*

The expansion of community involvement in the treatment and management of psychiatric patients, particularly as exemplified by the 1974 and 1982 reorganizations of the NHS, gradually changed the traditional psychiatric settings which had originally nurtured and supported clinical psychologists. Initially clinical psychologists had found themselves in psychiatric hospitals built in the nineteenth century away from centres of population. After the inauguration of the NHS, new psychiatric units were sited in general hospitals and local networks of support services were developed. As clinical psychologists became more involved in general hospitals and out-patient clinics as opposed to being used as an ancillary hospital provision of a department of psychiatry, the range of problems they were asked to deal with increased with consequent greater utilization of the many skills they possess to assist with various aspects of health care. Trethowan (1977) envisaged psychological services which would include commitment to primary health care and the development of preventive services.

Lamberts (1979) viewed primary health care as the boundary between the medical system and society. For most people, primary care means the first level of contact when seeking help from the NHS. In practice, the point of entry is usually through the GP who occupies a key position among the professional staff involved in primary health care. The other professionals most involved in primary health care are the health visitors, community nurses, treatment-room sisters, district midwives, and social workers. Pritchard (1978) in his *Manual of Primary Health Care* regarded health visitors, community nurses, treatment-room sisters, and district midwives as the main primary care team. Social workers were considered to be in a special relationship as their main concern is not health and clinical psychologists were listed among other professional staff, such as physiotherapist and occupational therapist, who may be included in a primary health care team under certain circumstances to offer specialist help. Psychological skills were deemed useful by Pritchard in the following conditions: agoraphobia and other phobic states, excessive dependence on psychotropic drugs, marital and sexual problems, excessive smoking and obesity, and intellectual deterioration after strokes and head injuries. In addition, the psychologist's training in group work was thought to be useful to help the primary care team to make group work effective. Rehabilitation work, particularly after injuries and strokes and the long-term care of the elderly, mentally handicapped, or other chronically ill in their homes, community or day hospitals have changed greatly with the involvement of clinical psychologists (see other chapters in Parts II and II.)

## GENERAL PRACTICE AND COMMUNITY CLINICAL PSYCHOLOGY

The movement of clinical psychologists from a hospital base into the community had undoubtedly been an important factor in redefining the profession. A great many discussions took place as to its feasibility, advisability, and morality. Kincey (1974), anticipating the first major reorganization of the NHS, made a cogently argued case for a closer liaison between GP and clinical psychologists. He suggested that clinical psychologists could be usefully employed on a 'peripatetic basis serving several practices or by attachment to health-centre teams'. The most compelling reasons given for this proposed change of location regarded the advantages of treating patients outside hospital, in the environment where problems had arisen (and were maintained), and the prophylactic value of psychological treatment at an early stage before hospital treatment had become necessary. His challenge was widely taken up, at least by clinical psychologists in the first instance.

Broadhurst (1977) published the results of a postal survey addressed to all clinical psychologists practising in the UK in 1975 and enquiring into their community involvement, particularly through general practitioners. Some 33 per cent or 216 completed questionnaires were received at the close of the survey. Among the respondents, the great majority were employed in psychiatric hospitals with a small number employed in general hospitals. There were also four clinical psychologists employed primarily to work with GPs, 30 worked both in a hospital and a community setting and 78 described their work as community orientated. Furthermore, the majority of respondents acknowledged that they were working with general practitioners, with medical specialists other than psychiatrists and/or with other workers in the community.

The type of referrals received from GPs included 56.9 per cent for individual treatment of behaviour problems, 14.4 per cent for group treatment, and 38.4 per cent for individual assessment. Other requests were received for involvement in research (27.3 per cent), teaching (56.9 per cent), and consultation (34.3 per cent) on various related clinical matters. It was evident from the above survey that clinical psychologists had been largely responsible for initiating their community contact and, through these, had made a substantial contribution to the community. The community-involved psychologists found many advantages in their contacts with GPs such as early treatment, treatment in the natural environment without stigma of mental illness, increasing acceptance of psychological models for behaviour disorders and ease of communication with GPs. Another survey carried out a year later and addressing itself directly to GPs of the Croydon Area Health Authority showed that there was considerable support among the GPs surveyed for having direct access to psychological services (Davidson, 1977).

In a study investigating GP and clinical psychologist agreement in their respective evaluation of the degree of psychological involvement seen in problems presented in two group medical practices, it was estimated that 8.4 per cent of the total population which consulted the GPs could benefit from referral to a clinical psychologist (McPherson and Feldman, 1977). Although the GPs were more likely to see a greater need for the psychologist's intervention than the clinical psychologist, there was a high level of agreement between them regarding the relevance of psychological factors in the cases they examined. The majority of problems which were encountered during the study as likely to be helped by a clinical psychologist were those involving anxiety and depression, insomnia, obesity, excessive use of alcohol, marital and sexual problems, and child and elderly person management. McPherson and Feldman concluded from their experience, that if their findings were extrapolated nationally, this would necessitate a threefold increase in the number of clinical psychologists to meet the potential primary care demand. In view of this, they made a number of suggestions designed to maximize effectiveness such as careful selection of patients, teaching other professionals or the families of certain client groups, as well as treating similar clients in groups. Other pleas for restraint and for the careful monitoring and evaluation of GP–clinical psychologist relationships in the wider context of NHS psychological services ensued (Hood, 1979; McPherson, 1981; Eastman and McPherson, 1982).

## EVALUATION

Evaluation of such a complex set of relationships, as is involved when assessments of clinical psychologists working in primary health care are made, is not an easy task and benefits are unlikely to be spread evenly among all participants. McPherson (1981) reviewed assessments made of the contribution of clinical psychologists to primary care by attempting to identify the advantages which had accrued for the various parties involved such as patients, the NHS, GPs, and for clinical psychologists themselves. Various conclusions can be drawn from the tentative data available and, until there is more concrete evidence of quantifiable benefits, there is no doubt that the evidence will be used to back up different positions regarding the main issue of whether or not psychologists should be seen to work in primary health care. As things stand, it would also be wrong to underestimate the strong feelings among certain clinical psychologists, GPs, and patients that the enterprise had been successful and valued. While it is too early to be able to give definitive answers on all aspects of the contribution of clinical psychologists to primary care (or otherwise), at least it can be said that a salutary climate in favour of such evaluations has permeated this area of psychological practice from the start. It is hoped that cost/benefit issues will be pursued with equal vigour in other areas where clinical psychologists have involved themselves. As long as clinical psychologists remain a numerically small group, one service or other will be undermanned. Who is to say that one client group is more deserving than another?

## SITING OF PRIMARY HEALTH CARE SERVICES

The most suitable location for clinical psychologists in primary care has been a matter for concern and has depended largely on the local conditions individual psychologists found themselves in. It would seem at first glance that a mental hospital sited some distance away from its nearest town is unlikely to attract referrals from any other source than psychiatrists. However, Broadhurst (1977) found that psychologists working from mental illness hospitals had been able to contribute to primary care as well as their colleagues in general hospitals. For a number of clinical psychologists who wished to hasten the process of direct and close collaboration with GPs, as well as with other members of primary health care teams, the solution was to follow the model suggested by Kincey (1974) and to attach themselves to one or a small number of related GP group practices on a sessional basis (Johnston, 1977, 1978; Kat, 1978; Ives, 1979; Koch, 1979; Earll and Kincey, 1980; Spector, 1980). There is no doubt that, through their pioneering efforts, the above (and many others who followed similar leads) have been instrumental in demonstrating the capability of clinical psychologists to make valid and sustained contributions in primary health care settings.

Another group of clinical psychologists who had developed a service in a health centre without GPs and wished to attract referrals from them fared less well initially (Hallam and Liddell, 1978; Liddell *et al.*, 1981). It was not until after they had contacted their District GPs individually to describe their service that they started to receive the referrals they had hoped to stimulate. One reason for their initial lack of success seemed to be that the GPs of the District had not been in the habit of dealing with clinical psychologists in the past and consequently appeared hesitant to entrust their patients to people whose qualifications, training, and skills were something of an enigma to them. On the other hand, the GPs in question were found to be very approachable and interested once contacted and 69 per cent of the total number of GPs in that District made time available to speak with the clinical psychologist who had contacted them. As a result of these contacts, a substantial and steady flow of GP referrals was subsequently received at that particular clinic. In addition, other members of local primary health care teams such as community nurses, health visitors, and social workers also sent referrals and, on a number of occasions, phoned for advice in regard to particular patients they were responsible for.

From the above experience, it was evident that GPs varied a great deal in the degree of psychological involvement they perceived in their surgeries and/or willingness to refer their patients. In a follow-up study conducted some two and a half years after individual GP contacts were made, it was found that 38 per cent of the contacted GPs (scattered over 21 practices) had referred between one and ten of their patients and that over 50 per cent of the total referrals came from *three* of these practices (Liddell *et al.*, 1982). Eastman and McPherson (1982) also found great variation when they interviewed a sample of 30 GPs in the West Midlands regarding their perception of psychological problems. Kat (1981), having taken as a theme the processes of Primary Health Care in the NHS, pointed to the vagaries in general utilization of health services and the complex explanations given for this phenomenon which included the involvement of social and psychological factors in addition to epidemiological ones. He observed that 'activities of general practice — consultations, visits, etc. cannot be used as a measure of morbidity' because it cannot be presumed that referral and illness are perfectly correlated. In view of these known variations, it would seem that clinical psychologists who are concerned with the provision of district services should think of locating themselves in a place which is accessible to all GPs and other primary health care professionals of their particular district rather than just a few practices. On the other hand, it is also hoped that salaried posts will be developed in some large GP practices or among smaller group practices who may like to join forces to employ such persons to complement their existing services. Such posts would certainly be welcomed by psychologists who wish to specialize in this type of setting and continue in its development and evaluation.

## CLINICAL PSYCHOLOGISTS ON PRIMARY HEALTH CARE TEAMS

Pritchard (1978) saw psychologists in a rather peripheral position in relation to primary health care teams but welcomed further considerations in the light of contributions made by them on some teams. The BPS was asked to provide evidence to the DHSS Joint Working Party on the Primary Health Care Team. In its report (BPS, 1979), it commented that, in practice, primary health care teams operated under different models and that such diverse and flexible organizations should be retained to meet local needs. It was also pointed out in the report that a variety of activities were included under the heading of primary health care, making the concept ill-defined and amorphous. For instance, under this generic term, activities with widely differing time perspectives and requiring different priorities in the workload of the different professions involved were included. At the time of the report, primary health care applied equally to acute and crisis oriented services, prevention oriented services, and services for those with long-term chronic problems. One of the most basic confusions was seen as the lack of distinction made between primary health care which is characterized as a generalist service and specialist care in the community. It was concluded that clinical psychologists were able to work in the generalist manner required in primary health care as well as the specialist manner they had adopted in the past, but that the potential demand for psychologists in the generalist role could not be realized without profound changes in the size and structure of the profession.

## PSYCHOLOGICAL PROBLEMS SEEN IN PRIMARY HEALTH CARE SETTINGS

In practice, there is fairly close agreement between clinical psychologists and their other professional colleagues regarding the type of problems, both acute and chronic, which are likely to benefit from a psychological approach. This agreement may be due in part to the increasing involvement of psychologists in the large number of areas of health care provided by the NHS. District based clinical psychologists were better able to demonstrate their skills, under such an arrangement, than they had been able to do under the constraints which necessarily operated when they were solely attached to departments of psychiatry. The increasing visibility psychologists gained through district appointments made them better understood and valued by more people than had been the case in the early days of their establishment in the NHS.

The classification of individual clinical problems offered by Kincey (1974) appeared just as relevant after almost 10 years of its publication. At the time, he offered the following framework for clinical problems with which psychologists could help in primary care settings: (1) problems of anxiety and stress, (2) habit disorders, (3) educational–occupational difficulties or decisions, (4) interpersonal–social–marital problems, (5) psychological adjustment to problems stemming from physical illness or other significant life events involving medical care. The above framework accommodated a wide range of clients, many of whom cannot be appropriately labelled mentally ill, therefore likely to be the province of psychologists more than psychiatrists, although they have been referred to both in the past. In view of this, the expansion of psychological services is likely to relieve some degree of pressure from psychiatrists whose numbers are acknowledged to be too small to supply the demand made on their expertise. Some of the concepts of mental illness were discussed earlier (see Chapter 5. It should also be pointed out that mental illness classifications have gone into several systematic revisions and that psychiatrists have been well aware of the deficiencies inherent in a system which classifies diseases rather than people. In the Ninth Revision of the International Classification of

Diseases (WHO, 1978) several welcomed changes were made, one of which was the addition of adjustment and stress reactions to the existing categories. It had become increasingly evident that the classical descriptions of neurosis and psychosis did not apply to a large number of individuals who presented with abnormal but transient states of emotional disturbance. Adjustment and stress reactions were described thus: (1) acute reaction to stress to apply to a transient state induced by severe mental or physical stress, and (2) adjustment reactions denote more prolonged reactions usually in response to stress of a less spectacular nature but of longer duration. Individuals suffering from these adjustment and stress reactions are less likely to be seen by their GPs in the first instance who are in turn often unwilling to refer these patients as 'psychiatric cases'.

## BEHAVIOURAL MEDICINE

Stress regarding physical illness is increasingly acknowledged as an important factor within medicine itself which is encouraged to adopt a biopsychosocial approach to replace the more rigid biophysical approach of previous generations (Engel, 1977; Lipowski, 1977). Rachman and Philips (1975), in a now classic book, took the initiative in Britain in demonstrating the contribution of psychology to medicine; other relevant books by British clinical psychologists followed (Vingoe, 1981; Griffiths, 1982) as well as publications of interventions in specific medical settings (Broome, 1980; Nichols, 1981). There is a growing feeling of optimism among clinical psychologists that the behavioural techniques which had been successful in the treatment of mental illness will be equally if not more successful in the field of general health care. Lang (1980) justified this optimism in the following way:

> Experimental behavioral psychology is primarily a psychology of the intact central nervous system and the neurochemically normal brain. The tradition of experimental psychology is the study of normal human beings and animals, in search of general principles which can explain and systematize all behavior. Thus, most of our information concerns how people in general learn, perceive, are motivated, and so forth. Instances of serious psychopathology represent deviations from the norm, which are by definition less readily predicted from our knowledge of human action and, indeed, represent inconsistencies with the principles of behavior in which psychologists have confidence. Thus it is reasonable to expect that behavior modification methods will be more effective with the psychologically normal individual (who happens to be suffering from illness) than with people afflicted by a fundamental disturbance of behaviour. The application of behavioural engineering to such tasks as psychological preparation for surgery, encouraging behaviour consistent with disease prevention, or maintaining a drug regime is more straightforward, more within the bounds of present knowledge, than the cure of a serious psychological defect (Foreword, xviii).

Reading (1982), addressing himself to clinical psychologists in medical specialities other than psychiatry, advocated the development of group interventions, the use of ancillary staff, and the development and refinement of research methodologies including new measures of psychological states to meet the growing demand.

Matarazzo (1980) followed the development of behavioural health and health psychology from behavioural medicine. He offered the following definitions of behavioural health and health psychology:

> *Behavioral health* is an interdisciplinary field dedicated to promoting a philosophy of health that stresses *individual responsibility* in the application of behavioral and biomedical science knowledge and techniques to the *maintenance* of health and the *prevention* of illness and dysfunction by a variety of self-initiated individual or shared activities (p. 813).
> *Health psychology* is the aggregate of the specific educational, scientific, and professional contributions of the discipline of psychology to the promotion and maintenance of health, the prevention and treatment of illness, and the identification of etiologic and diagnostic correlates of health, illness, and related dysfunction (p. 815).

## CLINICAL PSYCHOLOGISTS IN THE SOCIAL SERVICES

During the 1970s posts for clinical psychologists were developed in social services departments. Brown (1981) examined the differences between social services departments and the other two state agencies which had employed professional psychologists in the past, namely the health service and the local education authorities. In his view, social services departments differ from the other two in that they employ less trained professionals of any description, they foster a generic training and mode of operation for social work, and the scope of their responsibilities is more extensive than either health or education since these responsibilities extend to the welfare of every individual from birth to death. In addition, the department of social services has not yet created a dominant professional group and most departments have still to find a satisfactory mode of operation.

Bender (1979) proposed a multi-level approach as a model of operation for psychologists in social services departments. The three main levels suggested by his model were:

1. Working with clients, either individually or in groups,
2. Working with staff in helping larger groups of clients,
3. Working with managers in monitoring, policy, and planning.

Examples of activities carried out at each of the above levels were given from the activities of a group of psychologists who have developed services in the same social services department during a period of over ten years. Other clinical psychologists have been in evidence in assisting social services departments with their services for children, the mentally ill, and the mentally handicapped (Brown, 1981; see previous relevant chapters).

Regarding care in the community, a recent DHSS document stated:

> Most people who need long-term care can and should be looked after in the community. This is what most of them want for themselves and what those responsible for their care believe to be the best (DHSS, 1981, p. 1).

The above document, although mainly concerned with the needs of elderly, mentally ill, and mentally handicapped people, also considered the physically disabled and the chronically sick for transfer to the care of social services departments. In view of this, one can only agree with Bender (1979) who concluded that — 'social services departments, with their very wide range of provisions, offer great opportunity for the development of *community psychology*' (p. 9).

## CONCLUDING COMMENTS

There has been a great deal of confusion regarding the nature of primary health care which has encompassed a variety of diversified activities carried out in the community.

Clinical psychologists have amply demonstrated their ability to contribute to acute or crisis intervention services as well as to those which cater for individuals who need long-term care and support in the community. Hopefully more prevention services will be developed including them in the future. In the view of their small numbers, it seems that they need to increase their effectiveness by using a combination of approaches and by being less case oriented than they have been in the past.

## REFERENCES

Bender, M. P. (1979). Community psychology: When? *Bulletin of The British Psychological Society,* **32**, 6–9.

British Psychological Society (1979). *Evidence to the DHSS Joint Working Group on the Primary Health Care Team.* Leicester: BPS.

Broadhurst, A. (1977). What part does general practice play in community clinical psychology? *Bulletin of The British Psychological Society,* **30**, 305–309.

Broome, A. K. (1980). Clinical psychology within obstetrics and gynaecology. *Bulletin of The British Psychological Society,* **33**, 357–359.

Brown, B. (1981). Constructing psychological services in social services. In I. McPherson and A. Sutton (eds), *Reconstructing Psychological Practice*. London: Croom Helm.

Davidson, A. F. (1977). Clinical psychology and general practice: A preliminary inquiry. *Bulletin of The British Psychological Society,* **30**, 337–338.

Department of Health and Social Security (1981). *Care in the Community: A Consultative Document on Moving Resources for Care in England.* London: DHSS.

Earll, L., and Kincey, J. (1980). Evaluation of psychological intervention at primary care level — a controlled trial. Paper presented at The British Psychological Society Conference, Aberdeen.

Eastman, C., and McPherson, I. (1982). As others see us: General practitioners' perceptions of psychological problems and the relevance of clinical psychology. *British Journal of Clinical Psychology,* **21**, 85–92.

Engel, G. L. (1977). The need for a new medical model: A challenge for biomedicine. *Science*, **196**, 129–136.

Griffiths, D. (ed.) (1982). *Psychology and Medicine*. London: BPS/MacMillan.

Hallam, R. S., and Liddell, A. (1978). A community clinic for teaching psychotherapy. *Bulletin of The British Psychological Society,* **31**, 145–146.

Hood, J. E. (1979). Clinical psychology and primary care: A plea for restraint. *Bulletin of The British Psychological Society,* **32**, 422–423.

Ives, G. (1979). Psychological treatment in general practice. *Journal of The Royal College of General Practitioners,* **29**, 343–351.

Johnston, M. (1977). The treatment of agoraphobia in general practice. *Behavioural Psychotherapy,* **5**, 103–109.

Johnston, M. (1978). The work of a clinical psychologist in primary care. *Journal of The Royal College of General Practitioners,* **28**, 661–667.

Kat, B. (1978). Primary health care: On finding one's place in the team. *Bulletin of The British Psychological Society,* **31**, 154–156.

Kat, B. (1981). The processes of primary health care. Paper presented at the West Midlands Branch of the DCP Symposium 'The Why, What and How of Psychology and Primary Care', Worcester.

Kincey, J. (1974). General practice and clinical psychology — some arguments for a closer liaison. *Journal of The Royal College of General Practitioners,* **24**, 882–888.

Koch, H. C. H. (1979). Evaluation of behaviour therapy intervention in general practice. *Journal of The Royal College of General Practitioners,* **29**, 337–340.

Lamberts, H. (1979). Problem behaviour in primary health care. *Journal of The Royal College of General Practitioners,* **29**, 331–335.

Lang, P. J. (1980). Foreword. In B. Melamed and L. J. Siegel (eds), *Behavioral Medicine: Practical Applications in Health Care.* New York: Springer.

Liddell, A., May, B., Boyle, M., and Baker, M. (1981). How to stimulate GP referrals to a clinical psychology unit. *Bulletin of The British Psychological Society,* **34**, 164–165.

Liddell, A., May, B., Boyle, M., Baker, M., and Hughes, M. (1982). GP satisfaction with a clinical psychology unit service. *DCP Newsletter,* **No. 37**, 21–24.

Lipowski, Z. J. (1977). Psychosomatic medicine in the seventies: An overview. *American Journal of Psychiatry,* **134**, 233–234.

McPherson, I., and Feldman, M. P. (1977). A preliminary investigation of the role of the clinical psychologist in the primary care setting. *Bulletin of The British Psychological Society,* **30**, 342–346.

McPherson, I. (1981). Clinical psychology in primary health care: Development or diversion? In I. McPherson and A. Sutton (eds), *Reconstructing Psychological Practice.* London: Croom Helm.

Matarazzo, J. D. (1980). Behavior health and behavioral medicine: Frontiers for a new health psychology. *American Psychologist,* **35**, 807–817.

Nichols, K. (1981). Psychological care in general hospitals. *Bulletin of The British Psychological Society,* **34**, 90–94.

Pritchard, P. (1978). *Manual of Primary Health Care: Its Nature and Organization.* Oxford: Oxford University Press.

Rachman, S. J., and Philips, C. (1975). *Psychology and Medicine.* London: Maurice Temple Smith. (2nd ed, 1978, Harmondsworth: Pelican).

Reading, A. E. (1982). Strategic and methodological aspects of behavioural medicine. *British Journal of Clinical Psychology,* **21**, 79–84.

Spector, J. (1980). An evaluation of clinical psychologists' involvement in primary care. Unpublished M.Sc. thesis, North East London Polytechnic.

Trethowan, W. H. (1977). *The Role of Psychologists in the Health Services*. London: HMSO.

Vingoe, F. J. (1981). *Clinical Psychology and Medicine: An Interdisciplinary Approach*. Oxford: Oxford University Press.

World Health Organization (1978). Glossary of mental disorders and guide to their classification. In *Manual of the International Statistical Classification of Diseases, Injuries and Causes of Death*, 9th ed. Geneva: WHO.

# *PART IV*

# Clinical Psychologists in Other Countries

The Practice of Clinical Psychology in Great Britain
Edited by A. Liddell


*Chapter 14*

# *Clinical psychology in other European countries*

*Karen Hassel*

It is impossible to do full justice to the title of this chapter. Continental Europe is far from a unity; it embraces many different countries all of which have their own history and culture as well as separate social, economic, and political systems. The disparities in the educational systems and in the organization of the professions involved in the health and social services of these countries contribute to the confusion. In view of this, the current status and activities of clinical psychologists practising in various continental European countries need to be related to each country's tradition in psychology and to its individual evolution of professional training.

The main focus of this chapter will be on the Scandinavian countries of Norway and Sweden. These countries have witnessed the most progressive legislative development concerning the professionalization of psychology in Europe (Fichter and Wittchen, 1980). The other countries of Scandinavia will be viewed in relation to the above and from this northern perspective other countries, both in Western Europe and in the socialist countries of eastern Europe, will be highlighted.

## SCANDINAVIA

### Norway

The first psychological institute at the University of Oslo was founded in 1909. The first professor of psychiatry, Ragnar Vogt, later got the honour to be referred to by Sigmund Freud who stated that the first mention made of psychoanalysis in a textbook of psychiatry was made in the Norwegian language. Professor Vogt's interest in psychoanalytic theories had an important impact on the development of Norwegian psychology. However, it was left to Harald Schjelderup, the first professor of psychology, to go beyond Vogt's theoretical interest into practically oriented psychoanalytic research. The first textbook of psychology to combine experimental and psychoanalytical thinking was Schjelderup's *Psykologi* published in 1927. This book is still considered relevant today. In the 1930s, Norwegian psychology received valuable inspiration from the country's refugees. Perhaps the one to have had the greatest influence was Wilhelm Reich with his 'character analysis'. Otto Fenichel was also to be found amongst many other well known personalities who lived in Norway for a while.

In the 1920s a heated debate regarding psychoanalytic theory and practice had been conducted and it was to reach its height during Reich's stay. This debate culminated in a royal resolution that limited the right to use psychoanalytic methods for diagnosis and psychotherapy. Four psychologists were among those who got the authorization, and with this it was stated that those other than medical doctors were qualified to practise psychoanalysis (Skard, 1959). During the Second World War the University was closed (1943–45); nevertheless, plans for a new and more practically oriented discipline were developed and progress in this direction continued until the present day.

*Education and training.* The training of psychologists is carried out at the Psychological Institute of the University of Oslo and in the Faculty of Psychology of the University of Bergen. Both universities have similar systems but their training is slightly different. Training programmes are frequently revised to take into account the requirements of the Psychology Act (see below).

A national professional council for psychology, which includes representatives from all institutions teaching psychology at university level, has worked out standard criteria for the Norwegian degree in psychology (*embetseksamen*). These criteria serve as common guidelines for the university programmes. The following areas must be studied by the prospective psychologist:

1. factors (biological, intrapsychic, social, and economic) which regulate feelings, contact and communication between individuals and groups and those which prevent normal growth and adjustment;
2. certain professional skills and assessment techniques and their relevant application in various forms of psychological practice;
3. the set of rules and regulations regarding professional practice and personal conduct;
4. the basis of the psychologist's work and his/her function in society.

At the University of Bergen, the student starts with *grunnfageksamen* (2–3 terms) which is a general theoretical introduction to psychology. This stage does not qualify individuals for professional practice.

The psychological *embetsstudium* (cand. psychol.) has two parts, each normally taking two and half years of study. Each part is evaluated by a written report. The first part covers further theoretical and methodological study in the basic areas of psychology and in its most important supporting disciplines. Required laboratory courses or some form of field work complements the theoretical aspect, supporting the view that theory divorced from practice is of limited value. All teachers responsible for training in the first part of the course are specialist and carry out research in their respective fields. It is therefore left to them to decide the essential knowledge and experience which is useful to the students. The second part of the course is a generically oriented practical training which prepares students for professional work. This applied part is subdivided into five terms which cover both academic teaching and clinical experience:

Term 1. Teaching is given on clinical diagnosis and other professional skills, partly in psychiatric hospitals and partly at the university psychological clinics. Teaching regarding special education is also given along with two weeks' experience in a residential setting for special education.

Term 2. In addition to those in the first term, the students are given courses in learning problems, educational–psychological diagnosis and counselling. During this term, students are given a three-week practicum in a school psychology department.

Term 3. As the course progresses the students are introduced to clients which they treat under the supervision of qualified staff. Academic teaching covers psychopharmacology, milieu therapy, clinical neuropsychology, industrial and organizational psychology; practical experience involves training in a psychiatric out-patient or in-patient setting (9 weeks).

Term 4. Teaching in clinical community psychology, in research in psychotherapy, organizational psychology, and in school sociology is provided; practical experience is obtained at a neuropsychological clinic.

Term 5. There is no formal course work during this stage; the students finish a dissertation and prepare themselves for the final examination.

All psychologists thus qualified are allowed to do clinical and psychotherapeutic work. Trainees working in health institutions receive supervision of their clinical work (two hours per week) during their first two years. The Norwegian Psychological Association arranges different seminars as part of postgraduate training, but the clinical training takes place partly in psychiatric institutions and partly in psychotherapeutic and psychoanalytic institutions or associations. The Norwegian Psychoanalytic Institute and the Institute of Psychotherapy receive state support for their postgraduate programmes.

The Norwegian Psychological Association accredits specialists in clinical psychology. The requirements for the specializations are five years of clinical practice in at least two different institutions, with at least two of the five years spent as a full-time employee in the same institution. Furthermore, a minimum of two years must be spent under the supervision of a specialist with compulsory attendance at several postgraduate seminars.

*The professional role.* As a result of the Psychology Act of 9th March 1973, professional psychology in Norway entered a new era. In accordance with the Act a degree from a Norwegian university (cand. psychol.) became the basic qualification for a psychologist. The universities are now legally bound to implement the minimum standards required by the Act in their psychology training programmes. They must develop curricula and types of evaluation which enable their graduates to fulfil the role legalized by the Act. The Act also protects the use of the professional title 'psychologist', and theoretically enables restrictions to be placed on the use of various psychological methods and treatments and legislates on the limits of confidentiality.

**Sweden**

In Sweden the development from an almost pure academic position to an acknowledged profession occurred very rapidly. As late as 1958, a plan for the education of psychologists was implemented. This programme was on two levels, *fil. cand.* and *fil. lic.* the latter being a preparation for teaching and research. *Fil. cand.* did not qualify for independent psychological practice; it only allowed the graduate to carry out restricted psychological tasks such as assessment, which was the main psychological function at that time. Actually the *fil. lic*. was not a practical training either, and in order to develop as a clinician the *fil. cand.s* had to work independently and continue their own education in different ways, by practising and taking various courses of study.

In its 25 years of existence the Swedish Psychological Association had continually worked for better standards of education and for the legal recognition of psychologists. A new plan for the education of psychologists is currently in operation. There are still two levels of training; a basic education of three years in the university which was introduced in 1969, and two further years instituted in 1972. This training leads to *psykologexamen*. Theoretical courses are combined with practical sessions giving experience in assessment, treatment and prevention. After a further year's work in an agency decided on by the *Socialstyrelsen* (Social Department), trainees are officially recognized as *Legitimerad Psykolog*. The fully qualified psychologist is then part of medical personnel and is responsible for his/her professional work to the *Socialstyrelsen.*

*Clinical tradition and development.* Sweden does not have the same psychotherapeutic traditions as Norway. Its psychotherapeutic developments can be described as waves that washed over the country and changed the landscape commencing with group psychotherapy in the 1960s (Sigrell, 1980). Perhaps because of the lack of established individual psychotherapeutic traditions, group psychotherapy based on psychodynamic theory was enormously popular. A group psychotherapy association was founded and group psychotherapy training was started. The next wave was a milieu therapeutic one, and in its wake a family-therapy wave emerged, followed by approaches based on communication and systems theories. Later, other psychotherapeutic approaches made their appearance — psychodrama, *Gestalt* therapy, behaviour therapy, bioenergetics, and so on. In recent years Scandinavian associations representing the latter two movements were created.

Thus at the beginning of the 1970s psychotherapy predominated in Sweden. Still more separate associations started to organize their own training in therapy, not only in group and family therapies but also in individual therapy. Teachers were recruited from Stockholm as well as from the UK and the USA.

In some of these years, Scandinavia found itself almost overflowing with American therapists offering seminars and different therapy training programmes. This led, especially in Sweden, to a concern about family therapy and politics. The apolitical stance of American therapists, whose ideas and methods were having such a strong impact on Scandinavians, was criticized. A politically-aware family therapy was demanded (Kjellquist, 1977).

*Postgraduate training in psychotherapy by the State.* In 1978 a proposal for postgraduate training in psychotherapy was accepted by the Swedish State. This training is open to all professions working with psychological problems. Requirements regarding former education, professional practice, and actual capacity to do psychotherapeutic work were specified. The training is organized in two stages: *Stage One* is an independent training of professionals who wish to broaden their knowledge and skills in their own field in order to include psychotherapeutic activities. In addition, it is the basic training for those who wish to continue to *Stage Two* which provides a thorough training in psychotherapy.

*Stage One* training is carried out over three terms and consists of seminars (240 hours), individual and/or group supervision (60 and 120 hours respectively), and personal therapy (group 120 hours, individual 50 hours). The candidates must have had three years clinical experience and have had the opportunity to practise therapy between *Stage One* and *Stage Two* training.

*Stage Two* prepares the students not only to practise but also to direct therapeutic activities and act as consultants in psychosocial activities and preventive work. The training in *Stage Two* lasts six terms and includes seminars (460 hours), individual supervision (100 hours) or supervision in group (200 hours), individual personal therapy (75 hours) or personal therapy in groups (160 hours). The students must be exposed to both forms of these activities.

The aim of this programme is to provide such a calibre of knowledge that is viewed, especially in *Stage Two* as equivalent to advance theoretical university education (Sylvander, 1980). Psychologists are the only professionals whose basic university course is accepted in place of *Stage One* education. All other existing training programmes in psychotherapy which are administered by the different groups and associations (some 50 programmes are in existence) are validated against this state programme.

**Denmark**

Denmark has the oldest psychological institute in the Nordic countries. The psychological laboratory was founded in 1894. Professor Lehman was the first professor of psychology (1910). A special version of phenomenological psychology developed by Professor Rubin has traditionally had a strong impact on clinical theory and thinking in Denmark. Three different university examinations prepare psychologists to practise. The training for *psykologisk kandidatexamen* (cand. psych.) aims to provide a background for independent psychological work; its emphasis is on breadth of subject matter and its duration five and a half years.

*Magisterkonferensen i psykologi* is primarily a training in research methods and few students take this examination. *Pedagogisk Kandidateksamen i psykologi* (cand. paed.) aims to train teachers to solve the problem of shortage of school psychologists. It normally takes 3½ to 4 years after qualifying as a teacher with a minimum of two years' teaching experience.

In the last years the Danish Psychological Association has established a postgraduate training programme. The programme is organized around the concept of basic groups of up to ten members. These groups aim to provide, under experienced leadership, peer supervision of clinical practice, discussion to plan clinical activities, and group directed academic tutorials. The participants in this scheme also receive at least six general courses, more formal teaching and five specialist courses (*Dansk Psykolognytt*, 1980). The training does not qualify for any recognized title or status. The Danish Psychological Association has approximately 1,500 members. One-third of the membership is employed in clinical psychology, as school psychologists, in hospitals, or in residential treatment homes. Since 1973 a new group of psychologists has emerged, namely psychologists without employment; 82 psychologists are unemployed and 193 occupy part-time posts (Bakdal, 1980).

**Finland**

This country did not produce special plans for the education of psychologists until 1980. Academically, psychology is placed as both a natural science and a humanistic and philosophical science. The Finnish Psychological Association exercises some sort of quality control by giving approval only to members who fulfil their requirements which is *fil. kand. examen* or an equivalent academic degree (similar to a Master's) this being the highest degree in psychology. In addition a minimum of three years' professional practice must be completed with between five and six special courses approved by the Association.

From 1980 a decree regarding psychological examination came into force. In accordance with this decree psychologists are required to follow 180 weeks of study which include 10 weeks in a practical setting. All Finnish universities follow the same framework for the education of psychologists and requirements are clearly specified. This new pattern of education appears less theoretical than previously but the more advanced parts of the programme still rely heavily on methods of psychological research and both practitioners and researchers are trained similarly.

### Iceland

The University of Reykjavik provides only an undergraduate programme in psychology. To obtain a higher degree the students have to go abroad, usually to Denmark. In 1979, the Nordic Psychological Congress was held in Reykjavik with Iceland's 50 psychologists acting as hosts. The congresses have been held every three years since 1947.

### Nordic co-operation

The Nordic Council (*Nordisk Råd*) approved as early as 1958, a recommendation regarding the legal recognition of psychologists. The governments of the countries involved were asked to consider such recognition, and the co-ordination of the guidelines regulating psychologists in all Nordic countries with a view to establishing a common labour market. In response to the Council's recommendation both Denmark and Sweden eventually concluded that problems relating to the standardization of training had to be solved before recognition was put forward. In Finland the registration of psychologists and the protection of the title Psychologist was proposed in the *Riksdagen* (Parliament) in 1969. The proposal was rejected but it was agreed that some legal regulation of the psychological profession was needed.

In 1980 a working party, appointed in 1976, reported back to the Council on the question of a common labour market for the social and medical professions. It was agreed that Norwegian and Swedish psychologists had equivalent qualifications as well as those Danes who have obtained the *cand. psych.* The question regarding Finnish training was postponed because it was difficult to assess the implications of their new plan mentioned above (Nu, 1979).

### Activities of the Clinical Psychologist in the Nordic Countries

In Sweden, as in Norway and many other countries, the pioneer clinical psychologists were found in child guidance clinics or similar settings. Hertzman-Ericson (1980) pointed out that in the 1940s the psychologist was primarily involved in testing and diagnosis, in the appraisal of the patients' degree of psychic disturbance and in the evaluation of their potential resources. The clinics were run with enthusiasm by psychologists who constituted a new group that was eager to learn and understand more about psychic disturbance. Early in this development, they were seen to introduce some form of supervision of their own group. In the 1950s alternative forms of treatments became the focus of their activities — play therapy, individual or group therapy as well as parent groups. The outstanding features of the 1960s were a great expansion of intern education and training along with the development of various methods and evaluation procedures. A shift occurred from out-patient treatment to milieu-therapy in kindergartens, in special therapeutic schools, or in treatment homes. The clinical psychologists were leading in this development. In the last decade family therapy has dominated, especially in Sweden where its many immigrants have presented new problems to be tackled.

The different psychiatric institutions were and are still partly dominated by medical thinking, with its consequent emphasis on diagnosis. The psychologist operating in that system offered a service to the medical doctors and to the psychiatrists in particular by assisting in the diagnosis of the disturbance. From the 1960s onwards this picture has gradually changed and psychologists are accepted as taking part in treatment; psychotherapy both individual and group, now constitutes an important part of the psychologist's work. Another important aspect is the training and supervision of ward personnel of the institution which appoints them. Evaluation and research, where these activities are carried out, are most often performed by psychologists and psychiatrists. Participation in administration and planning is also more common and more attractive for psychologists today than it was a few years ago.

Most of the psychologists holding clinical positions in the Nordic countries work in psychiatric institutions for children, adolescents and adults, and in multidisciplinary teams both outside and within these institutions. Increasingly more emphasis is laid on out-patient treatment. In Norway, the psychologist who has specialized in clinical psychology may head a psychiatric out-patient clinic for children and adolescents. Denmark has had a long tradition of psychologists as heads of treatment homes for children and adolescents.

In the Nordic countries all health services are free and under government control. It is possible to have private treatment but it is only in Norway that the psychologists (with a clinical speciality) are reimbursed by the national health insurance scheme when referral has been made by a medical doctor. The general political trend is to invest in preventive work and out-patient treatment, trying to keep people out of institutions. The old institutions with hundreds of patients are gradually being run down and the psychiatric health services are organized in smaller units. This trend implies a broadened perspective on psychiatric problems and demands a change in the various professional roles. The clinically trained psychologist seems very well equipped for this development. For example, in a large scale Swedish project, *Nackaprosjektet*, three psychiatric teams were established in an area of 70,000 inhabitants, outside Stockholm. This well funded project aimed to organize the complete adult psychiatric services, keeping to a minimum the need for hospitalization by developing various types of community support systems. The report of this work (Hoffman, 1978) showed that by virtue of both their theoretical and practical training the clinical psychologists adjusted easily to the different professional role required of them.

With the aforementioned development in psychiatric services, it is evident that there is no longer any definite demarcation between psychiatric services and preventive work, and psychiatry has gradually been redefined in psychological and social terms as much as in medical terms. Nevertheless, when decision-making and final responsibility are at issue, the medical perspective is still dominant in Norway, as well as in the other countries.

Clinically trained psychologists work in various institutions and services for handicapped children. In addition to the more traditional functions, they are also engaged in the integration of services for these individuals in the local community as well as being concerned with the political implication of these problems. Clinical psychologists are important contributors in family consultation centres as therapists, consultants, and as supervisors to other professional groups. Child welfare centres have a responsibility not only for the physical, but also the mental health of the children. Therefore, clinical psychologists aid the early detection of disturbances and the planning of preventive activities at different levels. Hitherto they were mostly part-time consultants, but new posts are being established. The same trend is found in general hospitals, in maternity clinics, in paediatric and many other wards. The contribution of the clinical psychologist is looked upon as a valuable one. Clinical neuropsychology is a relatively new subject, but it is expanding rapidly. Research in clinical psychology needs to be strengthened and the universities of Oslo and Bergen have established two institutes to stimulate and train in clinical psychological research.

In practice, many psychologists start their professional career, not as supervised psychologists in a protected professional milieu, but more often as the only psychologist in a district (primarily as a school psychologist), or as the only psychologist in an institution, or in Norway, as an isolated community psychologist. This trend, together with the investment in preventive psychiatric work in the community has, especially in Norway, led to a heated debate regarding the concept of clinical psychology and the demands for clinical specialization. The concept 'clinical' is a medical one. A specialization in psychological treatment is proposed to replace that in clinical psychology. In some ways this entails loosening the ties with medical tradition and hospital treatment, and establishing psychology on its own two feet as an independent discipline which offers alternative treatment outside hospital.

In conclusion, the university education offered in the Nordic countries includes both academic and professional training. Very briefly, it seems that Finland emphasizes basic research and theoretical training, while Denmark stresses practical professional work. In Sweden and Norway there seems to be a better balance between the two aspects of training.

## OTHER CONTINENTAL EUROPEAN COUNTRIES

When looking at the rest of continental Europe, the picture is less clear and generalizations are more difficult to make in view of the great diversities already mentioned. The Council of Europe published a report in 1978 about the role of the psychologist as a member of a medical team caring for adults, children, and adolescents (Study Report, European Public Health Committee, 1978).

A questionnaire was sent to the health authorities of the member states, but the data did not provide a clear picture. The number of psychologists actually employed in these services differed enormously. It is obvious that the statistics thus obtained must be related to the population of the countries, development of their services, training and experience of the psychologists, and whether in full or part-time employment. However, the general trend was that the demand for psychologists was higher than the number presently employed. The minimum period of formal training for registration or recognition as a psychologist ranged from 4 years in Luxembourg to 6½ to 7 years in Norway. Some countries (e.g. Cyprus, Malta) do not provide university training for psychologists and students need to go abroad, either to other European countries or to the USA and Canada. Nevertheless, most countries appear to have postgraduate programmes for clinical psychologists.

Psychologists are seen to carry out different functions depending on the position held. Assessment, different forms of therapy, counselling, consultation, education, and research are the main functions of the practising psychologists. Generally, psychologists have great autonomy within a multidisciplinary team.

The report from the Council of Europe ended with a resolution which was adopted by the Committee of Ministers in November 1978 at the 296th meeting of the Ministers' Deputies and was later approved by the member states. It was recommended that the governments concerned consider the principles mentioned in the appendix to the report (Resolution (78) 61) when adopting national legislation, regulation, and practices. The governments of the member states were also invited to inform the Secretary General of the Council of Europe, at five-yearly intervals, what action had been carried out in accordance with the resolution. This resolution and its approval should be seen as the first step towards standardizing training and the professional status of psychologists in Europe.

What was not apparent from the Council of Europe Study Report was the growth in the activities of some psychotherapeutic groups who adhere to more or less restricted theoretical systems. These groups arrange seminars within private associations and institutions that provide training programmes. Many of these 'missionary' therapists coming from the USA (in particular California), seemed to have moved from country to country in Europe after shortlived successes. On the other hand, some therapeutic approaches have shown more stability. The Swedish psychologist Bo Sigrell (1980) has speculated that such approaches endure, (1) when the psychotherapeutic method is theoretically well-founded (i.e. documented research exists), (2) when there is a well-established international organization with its own journals which publish both research and discussions on training, and (3) when the host country already has prominent psychotherapists who wish to encourage technical and theoretical expansion of their activities.

When training is properly established approval is sought for official status as a postgraduate specialization by the various national psychological associations; following this legal recognition is sought. As yet very few countries have achieved legal recognition; in many countries the psychological association has granted approval. For example, in Holland, psychologists wishing to work as psychotherapists must belong to their national psychological association; there the title 'psychologist' has been protected since 1971. Protection was granted in East Germany in 1967, in Portugal in 1972, and in Norway and Sweden in 1973 and 1978 respectively. Certification is being prepared in West Germany and Poland. Austria has had legislation regarding the function of psychologists since 1978 (Fichter and Wittchen, 1980).

## West Germany

Almost all expertise in psychology and psychiatry disappeared in Germany with the Second World War. Few of the psychologists have returned, for the war represented a complete break, especially for the dynamic approach to psychology.

West Germany is a federation of lands which accords great autonomy both to its school system and to the health services. Psychology as a subject in its own right was not fully introduced in German universities until 1950. This education varies a great deal in content, being partly dependent on the availability of teachers. It takes five years to get a postgraduate qualification (*Diplom Psycholog*). Schools of psychotherapy have developed postgraduate programmes of training lasting three years but these give no formal qualifications. Seen through Norwegian eyes (Ekern, 1980) psychologists who have received therapeutic training in Germany appear to be well educated at the theoretical level they choose, but they do not appear so flexible and skilled in practice. The Psychological Association suffers from psychologists identifying and working for their own interest groups rather than for the Association. The situation varies so much from one part of the country to the other that it is difficult for psychologists to work in a unified manner towards future registration and approval of training programmes. It is, however, expected that new legislation regulating therapeutic activities will be put forward in a few years' time. Until then, psychologists are allowed to carry out assessment and provide counselling but it is tacitly accepted that many of them practise therapy as well.

## France

In France, the university training of clinical psychologists takes five years. The specialization which is formally defined relates almost exclusively to psychodiagnostics. The qualification required for employment as a clinical psychologist in public hospitals or related institutions is laid down in Articles 2 and 3 of a Decree of December 1971 and by an Order of February 1972. The qualification of psychologist is awarded by the Secretariat of State for Universities.

The health authorities indicated to the Council of Europe that the number of psychologists on the labour market exceeds current demand. However, compared with Norway and Sweden, France actually has a smaller proportion of psychologists employed in psychiatric services per 100,000 inhabitants (2.5 and 2.6 compared to 2.3 respectively), and there is no reason to believe that the incidence of psychological problems is fewer. One explanation may be that psychologists in France are not allowed to be involved in treatment. However, it was acknowledged by many institutions that psychologists did practise psychotherapy. This is another example of the discrepancy between the official position regarding the function of psychologists and what in practice they do by obtaining qualifications through privately organized and financed post-graduate training.

### Belgium

To obtain employment as a psychologist, a university degree in psychology is usually sufficient. However, as the number of psychologists seeking employment increases, additional qualification (further specialized training) is required. The university qualification is usually a *licencié* in psychology and/or education involving four or five years of study. It is the basis for further specialization in clinical psychology without the granting of a special title. Rules governing psycho-medico-social centres and the School and Vocational Guidance Bureaux are more specific with respect to qualifications that can be reasonably required. In institutions certified by the Department of Public Health, psychologists take an active part in examination (psychometric and clinical), in discussion of diagnoses with the team and in the therapeutic provisions. Moreover, teams in which psychologists play a therapeutic role are becoming increasingly numerous. It often happens that the psychologist is better trained than the doctor for certain specialized forms of therapy. The psychologist may also contribute a therapeutic role in residential institutions where a group approach to treatment is prominent (Council of Europe, Working Paper, 1976).

### Italy

Traditionally, in Italy, psychology has either been a branch of philosophy or has belonged to the institute of education when related to children. Psychologists do not have a tradition in therapeutic work and have not achieved registration or protection of their interests. University training is similar to that of France; for this reason many students go to that country to pursue their education. In 1968, legislation provided for the incorporation of psychologists in psychiatric hospitals as well as mental health centre teams.

### East Germany

The German Democratic Republic was founded in 1949 and during the first half of the 1950s psychology was introduced at university level (Kossakowski,

1980). It planned to give particular weight to a solid theoretical and methodological basis for the training of students in professional work, chiefly in education, clinical work, and industry. The total period of study is five years and it is possible to specialize in clinical psychology during the last three years. This specialization is then acknowledged on the diploma. Advanced training in psychotherapy is also available to psychologists; behaviour therapy and client-centred therapy are the most important theoretical orientations of the university training programme (Fichter and Wittchen, 1980). The overall aims were to promote the development of psychology in theory and practice, to raise standards and support the development of humanist psychology at an international level. When the activities of the clinical psychologists practising in the GDR are examined, they reflect the development of the society in general. As Kossakowski stated, psychologists are involved with many others in the promotion of mental and physical health. In the health service system, psychologists deal with varied forms of diagnosis and carry out therapeutic work. In the last years, the preventive aspects of the psychologist's role have gained prominence when compared to psychotherapy. In addition, within the health service system and out-patients centres, clinical psychology is given a great part to play. What is less well known and different from Western European countries is the fact that clinical psychologists in East Germany along with engineering and industrial psychologists work directly in industry and the transport system. Their activities extend from participating in the construction of industrial plants and other work settings, through the creation of effective communication and management channels within the firm, analysis of problems delaying production (including those relating to strain and tiredness), and their solution up to advising the management regarding personnel selection. Psychologists are also gaining more influence in the forensic area by assessment, and involvement in the re-education and reintegration of offenders in society.

## REFERENCES


Bakdal, B. (1980). Psykologers arbejdsområder. *Dansk Psykolog Nyt,* **34**, 644–646.

Council of Europe (1976). Working papers and private notes to the working groups on the Study report.

*Dansk Psykolog Nyt,* **34**, 483–484 (1980). Information om Dansk Psykologforenings systematiserende efteruddannelse.

Ekern, S. (1980). Erfaringer fra en tysk praksis. *Tidsskrift for Norsk Psykologforening,* **17**, 361–364.

Fichter, M. M., and Wittchen, H. U. (1980). Clinical psychology and psychotherapy. A survey of the present state of professionalization in 23 countries. *American Psychologist*, **35**, 16–25.

Hertzman-Ericson, M. (1980). Från testing til hemma-hos-terapi. *Psykolognytt*, **22**, 15–16.

Hoffman, J. (1978). Psykologrollen inom Nackaprosjektet. In *Psykiatri i omvandling. Teamfunktion, personalroller och intern utbildningsverksamhet.* Appendix 5 to Spri rapport 7, Fack, 102 50 Stockholm.

Kjellquist, E. B. (1977). Familjeterapeuten — en konservativ politisk kraft? *Psykolognytt,* **8**, 4–7.
Kossakowski, A. (1980). Psychology in the German Democratic Republic. *American Psychologist*, **35**, No. 5, 450–460.
NU A (1979). Fri arbestmarknad inom hälso-ock sjukvården ock veterinär-väsenet. *Psykologer*, **24**, 119–132.
Sigrell, B. (1980). Psykoterapiämnet har fått fast forankring under 70-talet. *Psykolognytt*, **22**, 20–21.
Skard, Å. G. (1959), *Psykologi og psykologer i Norge*. Oslo, Universitetsforlaget.
Study Report (1978). *The role of the psychologist as a member of a medical team caring for parents, children and adolescents.* European Public Health Committee, Strasbourg.
Sylvander, I. (1980). Vårt arbete har varit detaljerat och noggrant. *Psykolognytt,* **15**, 8–10.

The Practice of Clinical Psychology in Great Britain
Edited by A. Liddell


*Chapter 15*

# *Clinical Psychology in the United States of America*

*Sol L. Garfield*

Clinical psychology has probably developed more rapidly in the United States than in most other countries. The most rapid growth has occurred since the end of the Second World War, when a variety of social and governmental factors contributed to this expansion. It will be worthwhile, therefore, to briefly review some of these developments as a background for understanding the current situation in clinical psychology in the United States.

## HISTORICAL INTRODUCTION

Clinical psychology in the United States is generally thought to have begun with the work of Lightner Witmer. Witmer, after receiving his Ph.D. degree under Wundt in 1892, was appointed director of the laboratory of psychology at the University of Pennsylvania. Four years later, in 1896, Witmer founded the first psychological clinic in the US, and gave the first course in clinical psychology. In fact, it was Witmer who named this area of psychology 'clinical psychology'. It would seem, therefore, that he is rightfully viewed as the founder of clinical psychology. A more detailed description of Witmer's contributions can be found elsewhere (Garfield, 1965, 1974). However, it is worth mentioning also that Witmer founded, edited, and wrote for the journal, *The Psychological Clinic*, from 1907 to 1935, at which time the publication of the journal ceased.

In spite of Witmer's contributions, his impact was surprisingly limited. Psychology was still in its infancy and there did not appear to be strong demands for psychological services. A more significant development, however, was also occurring around the turn of the century which was to have a greater impact on clinical psychology. This was the development of the mental age scale by Binet and his colleague, Simon, in France. The availability of a potentially worthwhile test of mental ability was of some consequence for those working with a variety of children's problems. The American psychologist, Henry Goddard, revised the scale for use in the US in 1908 and helped to popularize it. The first child guidance clinic was founded in Chicago in 1909, and the director, the psychiatrist William Healy, was much interested in the appraisal of mental abilities. The use of psychological tests was thus associated quite early with the development of clinical psychology.

A few other early developments can be mentioned before going on to more recent history. Although the first child guidance clinic in Chicago employed a psychologist, Grace Fernald, and thus provided a model for the employment of clinical psychologists, the number of such clinics increased very slowly. In a similar fashion, the development of the mental hygiene movement in the US and of psychoanalysis abroad had little immediate impact on the growth of clinical psychology in this early period, although they did at later periods. The Stanford-Revision of the Binet–Simon Scale by Lewis Terman and his colleagues at Stanford University in 1916 was an event of some importance. It was for many years the most recognized psychological test, and the hallmark of the clinical psychologist.

Thus, during the first three decades of this century and continuing through the fourth decade, clinical psychology was a very small and slowly developing field within psychology. Clinical psychologists were employed in child guidance clinics, institutions for the mentally retarded, a small number of state mental hospitals, and in universities. There were no legal standards or requirements in order to function as a clinical psychologist, and there were no special or organized training programmes in clinical psychology in the universities. The primary duties of the clinical psychologist centred around the administration of psychological tests, with a major emphasis on the Stanford–Binet Scale of Intelligence. A survey by Louttit (1939) of 111 psychologists in child guidance clinics indicated that 'psychometrics' was their most frequent activity, with over 86 per cent of the group engaged in this activity. Educational guidance and vocational guidance were the next most frequent activities. Psychotherapy, the currently most popular activity of psychologists in the US, was listed as the sixth most frequent activity. It should be noted also that clinical psychologists during this period were to a large extent professionally involved in working with children.

The advent of the Second World War changed matters drastically. There was an initial need for psychologists to help in the screening and selection of men for the armed forces. As the war continued and the battle casualties increased, there was a shortage of trained psychiatrists to provide the necessary diagnostic and treatment services. As a result, clinical psychologists were offered commissions as officers in the US Army in 1944, a special five-week course of training was provided, and clinical psychologists were assigned to military hospitals and medical units. Of importance here was the opportunity for a number of clinical psychologists to participate in a wider variety of activities with patients than previously, particularly individual and group psychotherapy.

When the war was over, the Veterans Administration (VA) had to deal with a large number of emotionally disturbed individuals who required a variety of in-patient and out-patient services. This agency, like the army, also sought the help of clinical psychologists. Positions were set up for clinical psychologists which, patterned after the military, mentioned such primary functions as diagnostic testing, research, and psychotherapy with appropriate supervision. This, therefore, provided a number of new and relatively well-paid positions for clinical psychologists. At first, positions were available for psychologists without the doctorate. However, in the latter part of 1951, the VA, in line with other developments to be discussed shortly, decided to require the Ph.D. degree for all clinical psychology staff positions.

Although there was a great need for clinical psychologists at this time, there were too few trained psychologists available for employment. The VA, therefore, in co-operation with qualified universities, set up a collaborative training programme. The essence of the programme was as follows: Graduate students admitted to the programme would spend approximately half a week at various VA installations. This would provide them with a stipend to defray the costs of graduate training as well as with clinical experience under supervision in VA hospitals and clinics. University faculty members would serve as consultants to provide instruction and liaison with the field settings. On the whole, the programme was successful and helped train a large number of clinical psychologists, a significant percentage of whom later took positions with the VA. For many years, over 700 students per year participated in the programme and the VA became the largest single employer of clinical psychologists.

At least three other developments during the immediate post-war period also deserve mention. Because of the shortage of personnel in the basic mental health professions — psychiatry, clinical psychology, psychiatric social work, and psychiatric nursing — the US Public Health Service and its National Institute of Mental Health also provided substantial support for graduate training in clinical psychology. Fellowships for students were provided, as well as funds for faculty salaries, equipment, and the like.

The other two developments pertain to events within the American Psychological Association (APA). The first was a decision in 1945 that both applied and scientific psychology should be in one organization with special divisions to reflect the various interests. Consequently, the American Association of Applied Psychology, formed in 1937, was disbanded and incorporated into APA, and the former's journal, the *Journal of Consulting Psychology* eventually became the clinical journal of the APA.

The other development of importance pertains to decisions reached concerning the training of clinical psychologists. In part, because of the demand from governmental agencies to indicate acceptable university programmes for possible support, the APA decided to implement a programme of accrediting doctoral programmes in clinical psychology. Also, in order to provide adequate guidelines for training, a Committee on Training in Clinical Psychology was appointed and an important report was issued in 1947 (American Psychological Association, 1947). The recommendations were subsequently discussed at a major conference on training held in Boulder, Colorado, in 1949 (Raimy, 1950). The conference provided a general definition and framework for clinical psychology in the US, as well as general guidelines for graduate training which have been of great importance in the subsequent development of clinical psychology.

Very briefly, the significant recommendations of the Boulder Conference were as follows. It was decided that the training programme would be a Ph.D. programme and that the clinical psychologist would be trained both as a scientist and as a practitioner. He was to be a psychologist first, and a clinician second. His training and expertise in research would constitute the unique contribution of the clinical psychologist to the mental health field. For the first time, also, a one-year internship was to become a required part of the programme.

By 1950, therefore, the situation as regards clinical psychology had changed rather markedly from what it had been in the pre-war period. Clinical psychology was recognized more clearly as a distinct speciality within psychology with specific training requirements; training for clinical psychologists had expanded greatly and was being partially supported by agencies of the federal government; there were abundant job opportunities available; and many individuals were interested in becoming clinical psychologists.

## FUNCTIONS AND ACTIVITIES

Deriving from the developments described earlier, the main professional functions of the clinical psychologist became crystallized as 'Diagnostic Testing, Psychotherapy, and Research'. Of these, diagnostic testing and research had links with traditional aspects of psychology, even though the approach to diagnostic testing was very different from what it had been in the past. Psychotherapy, however, was a relatively more recent activity and the one activity that led to conflicts with organized psychiatry — however, more about this later.

The diagnostic testing which became popular in the post-war era was influenced greatly by the work of David Rapaport and his colleagues (Rapaport *et al.*, 1945), and differed noticeably from the earlier emphasis on psychometrics. A comprehensive battery of tests was used which included the Wechsler-Bellevue Scale, the Rorschach, and several others. Not only was the test battery lengthy and complex, but the responses of the client or patient were viewed and interpreted within a framework of psychodynamic theory. This type of diagnostic testing was perceived as a highly skilled professional activity by both clinical psychologists and psychiatrists and was the primary activity of the clinical psychologist during this period. Projective techniques, regarded as a means of securing cues to unconscious conflicts and personality processes, were highly valued techniques and basic courses on the Rorschach method were introduced in most universities with graduate clinical programmes.

In the immediate post-war period, psychologists also participated to some extent in psychotherapeutic activities. The extent of this participation varied from setting to setting depending upon local ground rules and the particular participants involved. In some settings clinical psychologists did not engage in psychotherapy and the latter was reserved for psychiatrists. In others, 'selected' cases might be assigned to the psychologists, and in some instances, certain psychologists might be allowed to engage in psychotherapy and others not. The official policy in the VA at that time was that clinical psychologists were qualified to work with less severe cases under psychiatric supervision. However, this policy was not followed very strictly in a large number of settings.

The third primary function of the clinical psychologist, research, has tended not to be engaged in as much by clinical psychologists as the other two functions. The possible reasons for this are undoubtedly varied, and in the absence of adequate data, can only be speculated upon. It would appear that a large number of clinical psychologists were primarily interested in clinical activities and much less interested in research endeavours, in spite of the importance attached to research in the scientist–practitioner model and in the training universities. Many students expressed interest in research to conform to university expectations, but once their doctoral research was completed, they were essentially not very much involved with it. In some instances, complaints were made by clinical psychologists that their training in research emphasized laboratory procedures, was divorced from clinical concerns, and was viewed mainly as a hurdle to be overcome. A number of others said that the demands of their clinical duties were such that there was no time available for any research endeavours. Whatever the reasons, it seems clear that research was engaged in correspondingly less than diagnostic and psychotherapeutic activities (Kelly, 1961; Garfield and Kurtz, 1976).

The three functions mentioned, however, remained as the more or less recognized functions of the clinical psychologist. Over the years, there did appear to be a number of other functions which also were engaged in by clinical psychologists. These included consultation to agencies, teaching of various kinds, supervision of psychologists and other professionals and non-professionals, and administration. As clinical psychology grew and developed in the post-war period, changes also occurred in the amount of time devoted to the various functions and to their relative importance.

As mentioned earlier, diagnostic testing and assessment was the primary activity of clinical psychologists in the 1940s and 1950s. However, by 1960, such activities had decreased in relative importance and psychotherapy had become the dominant activity (Kelly, 1961). This trend has continued as indicated in a survey of 855 members of the Division of Clinical Psychology of the APA conducted in the mid-1970s (Garfield and Kurtz, 1976). In this survey, the percentage of time devoted by this sample of clinical psychologists to individual psychotherapy, was 25.07 per cent. An additional 4.35 per cent of time was given over to group psychotherapy, and behaviour modification was listed by 2 per cent. Thus, over 31 per cent of the professional time of clinical psychologists was devoted to psychotherapeutic activities. The next two most frequent activities were teaching with 13.82 per cent and administration with 13.21 per cent. Diagnostic and assessment activities constituted the fourth most frequent activity with 9.79 per cent. Other areas which can be mentioned were: clinical supervision, 7.78 per cent; research, 7.04 per cent; community consultation, 5.23 per cent; scholarly writing, 3.77 per cent; and research supervision, 2.71 per cent.

As the foregoing indicates, there has been a decided shift in the time devoted to various professional activities by clinical psychologists over the past few decades. Psychotherapy, a field dominated in the past by psychiatrists and not a prime activity of psychologists historically, has become the major involvement of clinical psychologists. In fact, probably a very large number of individuals enter the field of clinical psychology in order to become psychotherapists. Testing, however, which has been a unique activity of psychologists, has diminished in relative importance. Accompanying the latter development has been what appears to be a gradual decrease in the emphasis on projective techniques and in the use of lengthy batteries of tests for diagnostic purposes. Thus, in a relatively short period of time, there has been an important reordering of the value hierarchy of activities in clinical psychology. These changes have also been reflected in graduate training programmes which have been modified accordingly. Courses in projective testing have been reduced, and courses and practica in psychotherapy have been introduced and expanded.

## WORK SETTINGS

Clinical psychologists have been employed in a variety of settings. In earlier periods of development, they were primarily involved with children in school settings, child guidance clinics, and institutions for the retarded. In more recent times, clinical psychologists have become more heavily involved in working with adults in psychiatric hospitals and out-patient clinics, in medical schools, in general hospitals, in community mental health centres, and in private practice. The institutional affiliation of the sample of clinical psychologists surveyed by Garfield and Kurtz (1976) is presented in Table 15.1. As can be noted there, approximately 35 per cent were employed in such institutional settings as psychiatric or general hospitals, out-patient clinics, or medical schools. An additional 30 per cent were employed in university settings, and just over 23 per cent were in private practice. A little over 11 per cent of the sample were employed in such settings as public schools, the federal government, juvenile correction centres, rehabilitation centres, state departments of mental health, and private corporations. It can be mentioned also that there were no significant differences between men and women in terms of institutional affiliation, and almost half of the sample indicated some part-time engagement in private practice.

Although the great demand for clinical psychologists and other mental health professionals has diminished in recent years, with the exception of academic positions, there are still a variety of job opportunities available.

## CURRENT DEVELOPMENTS IN TRAINING

As indicated earlier, American clinical psychology adhered exclusively to the

TABLE 15.1 Primary institutional affiliations. Garfield and Kurtz, *American Psychologist*, 1976, **31**, p. 2. Copyright (1976) by the American Psychological Association, Reprinted by permission of the author

| Primary affilitation | *N* | % |
|---|---|---|
| None | 10 | 1.17 |
| Mental hospital | 72 | 8.42 |
| General hospital | 51 | 5.97 |
| Out-patient clinic | 44 | 5.15 |
| Community mental health centre | 64 | 7.48 |
| Medical school | 68 | 7.95 |
| Private practice | 199 | 23.27 |
| University psychology department | 188 | 21.99 |
| University, other | 60 | 7.02 |
| Other | 99 | 11.58 |
| Total | 855 | 100.00 |

scientist–practitioner model of training until around 1970. All graduate students were trained in both research and clinical skills. However, there was a certain amount of discontent expressed from time to time concerning this model by some clinicians who felt that their clinical training was inadequate, and by others who felt that their research training was also inadequate. There was an obvious conflict between scientific-research values and clinical ones that became more pronounced as the number of practising clinical psychologists increased in the post-war period. Some critics of the scientist–practitioner model claimed the model was an unrealistic one and that such conflicting or disparate goals could not be obtained. Others, however, argued that the model was a desirable one which had not been adequately implemented (Garfield, 1966).

The above-mentioned concerns were reflected in the appointment of a special APA committee to evaluate professional training (Committee on the Scientific and Professional Aims of Psychology, 1965), and in discussions held at a national conference on the professional preparation of psychologists in Chicago in 1965 (Hoch *et al.*, 1966). The report of the committee recommended consideration of alternative models such as more professionally oriented programmes leading to a Doctor of Psychology degree (Psy.D.) or to a Doctor of Psychotherapy degree. At the Chicago Conference several alternative models were introduced including the Psy.D. programme. However, the conference participants overwhelmingly reaffirmed their support for the scientist–practitioner model. Nevertheless, representatives from the University of Illinois stated their intention to seek university approval for setting up a Psy.D. programme in addition to their existing Ph.D. programme. Students would thus have a choice of models from which to choose. This actually did occur in a few years and a competing model was thus available (Peterson, 1968).

Not many universities have tended to follow the Illinois model. However, several other developments in training have occurred. Within a short time after the Psy.D. programme at Illinois was begun, a group of psychologists in the State of California, with the support of that state's psychological association, formed the California School of Professional Psychology. Unlike the Illinois programme, the school was a 'free standing' school and was not part of a department of psychology or affiliated with a university. The majority of the faculty were recruited on a part-time basis from practitioners in the community. Because of the demand on the part of prospective students for training in clinical psychology, and the fact that the approved university programmes can accept only a small percentage of those who apply, the California School has expanded rapidly to include four campuses in different parts of the state. It can be noted, too, that although the emphasis in on professional training, the degree awarded is the Ph.D.

At the present time there has been evident a decided growth in these non-traditional programmes. Three different patterns are discernible. The initial development of a Psy.D. programme along with the Ph.D. programme in a university department of psychology has not shown much growth or development. The Psy.D. programme at Illinois is actually being terminated since it apparently began to resemble increasingly the Ph.D. programme. A second pattern, currently evident at a few institutions is the professional school of psychology which is part of a university system and which is headed by a dean. These schools generally offer a Psy.D. degree in one or more professional areas of psychology with the Ph.D. given in a separate department of psychology, although there are variations in this pattern.

The third pattern of development is the most rapidly growing and potentially the most important of these recent developments. This is the marked increase in free standing schools of professional psychology. Such schools appear to be springing up all over the US. In California, alone, there were reported to be twenty-four such schools (Perry, 1979). Besides the increase in the number of such schools, the number admitted in many instances is much larger than that admitted to the university programmes. For example, the California School, may admit 100 new students at some of its campuses each year, whereas the average university programme admits eight to twelve new students. Such a development would appear to pose some potential problems with regard to the quality of training provided and to the definition and unity of clinical psychology in the US. Such concerns have been voiced in journal articles (Ericksen, 1966; Perry, 1979; Wollersheim, 1974) and at recent professional meetings. It is worth discussing some of these concerns.

Although professional programmes and schools were advocated and developed because of supposed limitations in professional training in academic programmes (Pottharst, 1970), a major concern expressed at present about these new programmes is precisely the same — concern over the quality of these programmes. These schools depend on students' tuition for practically all of their income, and this conceivably can influence standards for admission and retention in the programme. Part-time faculty are selected on a different basis than are full-time university faculty and are not as dependent on the programme as regular faculty since their main income is derived from their private practice or regular occupational setting. Undoubtedly, the standards among these schools vary considerably since local educational charters and accreditation procedures also vary. Since most of these schools have not sought or been granted accreditation by the APA, the actual data on the quality of the training programmes are lacking. This absence also causes concern.

Another major concern, expressed by the writer during a debate at a recent convention of the APA (Garfield, 1980a), pertains to the impact of these professional schools on the traditional definition of clinical psychology and what this may portend for the future of clinical psychology. As already indicated, clinical psychology under the scientist–practitioner model has grown and expanded enormously. In the last thirty-five years, the membership of the Division of Clinical Psychology in the APA has increased sevenfold and the number of approved training universities has quadrupled. During this period clinical psychology has become recognized as a vital profession in the mental health field. All of these developments would appear to be due at least in great part to the research oriented programmes of training received by clinical psychologists in the past. The development of non-university based professional programmes lacking the research training and emphases of traditional programmes is seen as posing a distinct threat to the acknowledged definition and uniqueness of clinical psychology as it has developed over the years. The development of purely professional schools has the clear potential of splitting the areas of research and practice within the field and of creating two different types of clinical psychologists with very different value systems. The existence of rival factions with opposite views could thus lead to the setting up of separate organizations and to some confusion concerning the definition of clinical psychology.

The present status of clinical psychology training in the US is thus in a state of flux which could have significant consequences for the future development of the field. It also is a reflection of a larger conflict in American psychology between scientifically and experimentally oriented psychologists on one hand, and practitioners, largely clinical psychologists in private practice on the other (Chein, 1966; Perry, 1979). This conflict, which has become intensified in recent years, will be discussed in more detail later.

## THEORETICAL ORIENTATIONS

Although clinical psychologists have indicated interests in a variety of theoretical views, certain orientations have been more preferred than others, and this also has varied over time. During the late 1940s and into the 1960s, psychoanalytic and psychodynamic theories were the most influential, and this emphasis was also manifested in university training programmes. This influenced both diagnostic and therapeutic practices. Psychodynamic long-term psychotherapy was highly valued as the most important and intensive form of therapy, whereas briefer and less evocative forms of therapy were viewed as palliative and supportive. In a similar fashion, projective techniques were considered a most important part of the psychologist's diagnostic testing battery since they were a means of tapping unconscious drives and conflicts. Even the more objective tests, such as the Wechsler Scales, could be interpreted from a psychodynamic orientation (Rapaport *et al*., 1945).

In the survey of clinical psychologists reported by Kelly in 1961, a psychoanalytic orientation was indicated by 19 per cent, a neo-Freudian by 13 per cent, and a Sullivanian by 9 per cent. Thus, 41 per cent of the sample clearly indicated a psychodynamic orientation. A preference for a learning theory orientation was expressed by approximately nine per cent, with four per cent expressing a preference for a Rogerian view. However, almost forty per cent of the sample identified themselves as eclectics.

In a more recent survey, the pattern of theoretical preferences appears to have undergone some change (Garfield and Kurtz, 1976). The total of the three psychodynamic preferences mentioned above was found to be 19 per cent in the later survey, thus indicating a noticeable decline. The preference for a learning theory orientation had increased slightly to approximately ten per cent. The preference for an eclectic orientation, however, has become the dominant one with almost fifty-five per cent of the sample indicating such a preference. Even some behaviour therapists are viewed, or view themselves, as eclectic behaviour therapists (Swan, 1979).

Thus, it appears that psychodynamic orientations among clinical psychologists have decreased over the past 15 or 20 years and that eclectic views appear to be the preference of slightly over half of the clinical psychologists surveyed. Although behaviour and learning theory oriented therapists are an exceedingly active and productive group of psychologists, they still are a relatively small group. However, some of their emphases and procedures undoubtedly have been utilized by other more eclectically oriented psychologists.

Another more recent development which can also be mentioned is the relative popularity of cognitive emphases in psychotherapy. Although Ellis's Rational-Emotive Therapy was listed by slightly less than two per cent of the sample in the survey by Garfield and Kurtz (1976), a number of other cognitive approaches and emphases have made their appearance in the recent literature (Bandura, 1977; Beck, 1976; Goldfried and Goldfried, 1975; Meichenbaum, 1977). There has also been evident a tendency on the part of some behaviour therapists to combine cognitive and behavioural components of therapy (Kendall and Hollon, 1979; Mahoney, 1974).

Recently, there have appeared also several books and articles which have discussed a *rapprochement* between psychodynamic and behavioural views (Birk and Brinkley-Birk, 1974; Feather and Rhoads, 1972; Marmor, 1971;

Marmor and Woods, 1980; Wachtel, 1977). Whether or not such divergent theoretical systems can be reconciled and integrated remains a debatable issue (Messer and Winokur, 1980). However, as previously noted there does appear to be a decided tendency toward espousing an eclectic perspective with correspondingly less reliance on more doctrinaire approaches (Garfield and Kurtz, 1976). It is perhaps no coincidence that two books with eclectic psychotherapy in their titles have appeared in 1980 (Garfield, 1980b; Palmer, 1980).

Although there has been evident a decided preference for an eclectic position in terms of the sample of clinical psychologists surveyed, the precise meaning or interpretation of the eclectic position is not at all clear. Although the term eclectic signifies that the person holding such a view does not adhere to one specific theoretical orientation, it does not allow us to know what views or practices eclectic clinical psychologists actually utilize. A study of 154 clinical psychologists, self-designated as eclectics in a previous survey, did indeed indicate they held a wide variety of views (Garfield and Kurtz, 1977). This was evident when they were asked to select the two theoretical orientations most characteristic of their eclectic views and the two orientations least characteristic of their views. These responses are presented in Table 15.2. In this analysis, learning theory was selected most frequently as a positive orientation, followed by psychoanalytic and neo-freudian orientations.

TABLE 15.2 Positive and negative responses to selected theoretical orientations. Garfield and Kurtz, *The Journal of Consulting and Clinical Psychology*, 1967, **45**, p. 79. Copyright (1977) by the American Psychological Association. Reprinted by permission of the author

| Orientation | Positive | Negative |
|---|---|---|
| Psychoanalytic | 46 | 41 |
| Neo-Freudian | 43 | 21 |
| Sullivanian | 24 | 16 |
| Rogerian | 36 | 25 |
| Learning theory | 72 | 26 |
| Existentialist | 17 | 44 |
| Humanistic | 29 | 16 |
| Rational-emotive | 18 | 57 |

In terms of negative reactions, the rational-emotive, existentialist, and psychoanalytic views received the most negative responses.

In the above-mentioned study, it was also of interest to see what were the most frequent combinations of the two orientations indicated by the respondents. As can be seen in Table 15.3, a number of combinations were selected, even though only those selected by five or more respondents are listed.

Actually thirty-two combinations were listed by the 145 respondents. The relative popularity of learning theory and the lack of popularity for the rational-emotive orientation in this sample is apparent.

TABLE 15.3 Combinations of theoretical orientations selected by five or more respondents. Garfield and Kurtz, *The Journal of Consulting and Clinical Psychologists*, 1977, **45**, p. 79. Copyright (1977) by the American Psychological Association. Reprinted by permission of the author.

| Orientation | n |
|---|---|
| Psychoanalytic and learning theory | 21 |
| Neo-Freudain and learning theory | 16 |
| Neo-Freudian and Rogerian | 9 |
| Learning theory and humanistic | 8 |
| Rogerian and learning theory | 8 |
| Psychoanalytic and Rogerian | 7 |
| Sullivanian and learning theory | 7 |
| Learning theory and rational-emotive | 7 |
| Psychoanalytic and neo-Freudian | 6 |
| Rogerian and humanistic | 5 |
| Sullivanian and humanistic | 5 |
| Psychoanalytic and humanistic | 5 |

The designation, eclectic, thus covers a wide variety of views and, by implication, of clinical practices. Two self-designated eclectics may actually hold somewhat opposing views. Nevertheless, the preference for an eclectic view does indicate a possible dissatisfaction with adhering solely to one theoretical orientation, and with the desire to select theories and methods which seem best for particular clients. Clearly, it represents a significant view in American clinical psychology.

## PROFESSIONAL ISSUES AND PROBLEMS

As clinical psychology in the US has grown and developed, particularly in the last thirty-five years or so, a variety of professional issues and problems have been encountered. Among the most important have been relationships with organized medicine and psychiatry, setting standards for professional practice, legislative efforts for certification and licensing, and value conflicts and power struggles within the APA and within clinical psychology itself. Because of space, only some of the most important items will be discussed.

As mentioned earlier, there was an association organized in 1937 to meet the needs of applied psychologists, the American Association of Applied Psychology (AAAP). It consisted of four sections, one of which was devoted to clinical psychology. Thus, there were two organizations, one for the science of psychology, and the other for the application of psychology. However, in 1945, the AAAP agreed to become incorporated into the APA as a sign of unity within American psychology, and thus both scientific and professional interests were henceforth to be represented by the APA. The latter in turn was to include divisions which would represent the various and diverse interests of psychologists in the US. Also, because of the growth of the APA, a central office was established in Washington, DC, with a full-time executive officer.

With the continued growth in the size of the APA and with the increase in professional concerns, the role and size of the central office has increased greatly. This expansion has also led to various types of conflicts. Clearly, there were differences in values between the traditional scientific and research emphases of psychology and the newer professional concerns for adequate training in clinical skills, for legislative activities, and for the less scientific and more intuitive emphases of the clinician. Such conflicts were evident in university departments of psychology as well as within the APA and state psychological associations. As the number of clinical psychologists increased more rapidly than did the number in other scientific specialities, various concerns were raised and there were skirmishes for power evident between the two groups. There were also verbal indications on the part of some psychologists of possible secession from the national organization. A group of experimental psychologists, for example, formed their own organization, the Psychonomic Society, in 1960. This group is still active today, has its own meetings, and publishes its own journals. The issues and conflicts are still apparent today and a resolution remains for the future. However, let us now proceed to some other developments which also were of some importance.

With the increase in professional activities, there was an obvious need to establish standards and codes of professional practice. Three important activities can be noted very briefly here. A profession or a speciality within a profession can set up some types of certification to specify competency in certain areas. Thus, following the model of medical specialities, an American Board of Professional Psychology (ABPP) was organized in 1947 to examine and certify psychologists in three areas of psychology — clinical psychology, counselling psychology, and industrial psychology. More recently, school psychology was added. Individuals with a Ph.D. and five years of experience are eligible to take the written and oral examination for the diploma in their speciality.

The ABPP diploma in clinical psychology, although a means of certifying a high level of competence in clinical psychology, was still a form of self-certification. Psychologists were also interested in legislation at the state level which would restrict the title of psychologist to those who reached at least a minimal level of training and experience. Securing state certification or licensure, however, was a more difficult goal to reach than was certification by the profession. In addition to the normal difficulties and hurdles usually encountered in getting bills enacted through the state legislatures and the governors' offices, there was strong opposition manifested by organized medical groups at the state and national levels. Most of the opposition appeared to be directed at the independent practice of psychotherapy, which the medical groups wanted to be under the control or supervision of physicians. Before discussing this problem further, however, it would be worthwhile to mention psychology's concerns and efforts with regard to ethical practice.

The APA, while insisting on the rights of its members to pursue their profession, devoted considerable thought to the issues involved in matters of independent practice. In 1953, a rather detailed code of ethics was finally published to guide professional practice and to ensure that adequate safeguards were observed in the practice of psychotherapy (American Psychological Association, 1953). For example, sections of the ethical code pertinent to these issues included the following:

> In clinical or consulting practice the psychologist must refer his client to an appropriate specialist when there is evidence of a difficulty with which the psychologist is not competent to deal (pp. 78–79).
>
> The psychologist who engages in psychotherapy is obligated to assist his client in obtaining professional help for all important aspects of his problem which fall outside the boundaries of the psychologist's competence. Most frequently this principle will require that adequate provision be made for the diagnosis and treatment of medical problems.
>
> (1) To this end, psychologists doing psychotherapy may be expected to establish and maintain effective inter-communication with a psychologically-oriented physician. The usual and most desirable interpretation of this principle is that the clinical psychologist will establish an effective working relationship with a psychiatrist. However, the principle is worded in more general terms in recognition of the fact that a psychiatrist may not be available, or that a physician with another speciality, such as pediatrics, may be more helpful in treating the medical problems of a particular client (pp. 79–80).

Psychologists thus took their new role and responsibilities seriously and did attempt to set up appropriate standards and safeguards. However, as indicated, there was decidedly strong opposition from medical groups. For example, a joint resolution was issued in 1954 by the American Medical Association, the American Psychiatric Association, and the American Psychoanalytic Association. This statement, among other things, emphasized the role of the physician in the diagnosis and treatment of 'illness that has chiefly mental symptoms'. They also stated that, 'Psychotherapy is a form of medical treatment and does not form the basis for a separate profession'.

Because of such opposition, certification and licensure proceeded slowly. By the end of 1955, only nine states had enacted such legislation. In New York State, a licensing bill for psychologists was passed by both houses of the legislature, but was vetoed by the Governor, primarily because of medical opposition. A certification act in New York finally was passed in 1956.

There is no need to retell the story of these conflicts and the struggle to secure legislative recognition for psychologists. It can simply be mentioned that by 1978, all fifty states in the US had enacted some type of legislation pertaining to psychology. Thus, approximately thirty-five years was required for legislation of this type to be secured. On the other hand, once this level of success was attained, a new problem emerged, namely, 'sunset laws'. In two states where the legislature recently reviewed existing legislation, the laws pertaining to the regulation of psychologists were rescinded. Concern has been expressed by psychologists in other states about the possibility of such legislative action in their states, but it is too early to know if such a pattern will occur elsewhere.

Although over the past thirty-five years there have been competitive skirmishes between psychology and psychiatry, and such incidents continue to occur with varying degrees of intensity, the relationship between the two professions is 'relatively' amicable. During this period of time, clinical psychology has not only grown and matured as a profession, but its stature as a significant profession in the mental health field has been increasingly recognized by governmental agencies and the public alike. Particularly in the area of mental health research clinical psychologists have played an increasingly significant role, and in the opinion of the author, this has given them a role which is not available to a purely service oriented profession.

## CONCLUDING COMMENTS

In the preceding pages, the author has attempted to provide an overview of clinical psychology as it has developed in the US. Because the field has developed so rapidly since the Second World War, the greatest emphasis has been devoted to this period. Attention was given to programmes of training, primary functions, theoretical orientations, work settings, and to professional problems and issues. The field of clinical psychology has experienced many changes and has faced a number of difficulties. Most of the latter have been successfully resolved, but new challenges and issues always appear to emerge. Currently, the issue concerning models of training appears to be an important one for the future of clinical psychology. How this will be resolved and in what directions clinical psychology in the US will move in the future cannot now be foretold.

## REFERENCES

American Psychological Association (1947). Committee on Training in Clinical Psychology. Recommended graduate training program in clinical psychology. *American Psychologist,* **2**, 539–558.

American Psychological Association (1953). *Ethical Standards of Psychologists.* Washington: APA.

Bandura, A. (1977). Self-efficacy: Towards a unifying theory of behavioral change. *Psychological Review,* **84**, 191–215.

Beck, A. T. (1976). *Cognitive Therapy and the Emotional Disorders.* New York: International Universities Press.

Birk, L., and Brinkley-Birk, A. W. (1974). Psychoanalysis and behavior therapy. *American Journal of Psychiatry,* **131**, 499–509.

Chein, I. (1966). Some sources of divisiveness among psychologists. *American Psychologist,* **21**, 333–342.

Committee on the Scientific and Professional Aims of Psychology (1965). Preliminary Report. *American Psychologist,* **20**, 95–100.

Ericksen, S. C. (1966). Responsibilities of psychological science to professional psychology. *American Psychologist,* **21**, 950–953.

Feather, B. W., and Rhoads, J. M. (1972). Psychodynamic behavior therapy. I. Theory and rationale. *Archives of General Psychiatry,* **26**, 496–502.

Garfield, S. L. (1965). Historical introduction. In B. B. Wolman (ed.), *Handbook of Clinical Psychology*. New York: McGraw-Hill.

Garfield, S. L. (1966). Clinical psychology and the search for identity. *American Psychologist,* **21**, 353–362.

Garfield, S. L. (1974). *Clinical Psychology: The Study of Personality and Behavior*. Chicago: Aldine.

Garfield, S. L. (1980a). Criteria for adequate psychology training: Do professional schools fit the bill? — the negative. Debate at the annual meeting of the American Psychological Association, Montreal, September 2.

Garfield, S. L. (1980b). *Psychotherapy. An Eclectic Approach*. New York: John Wiley.

Garfield, S. L., and Kurtz, R. (1976). Clinical psychologists in the 1970s *American Psychologist,* **31**, 1–9.

Garfield, S. L., and Kurtz, R. (1977). A study of eclectic views. *Journal of Consulting and Clinical Psychology,* **45**, 78–83.

Goldfried, M. R., and Goldfried, A. P. (1975). Cognitive change methods. In F. H. Kanfer and A. P. Goldstein (eds), *Helping People Change*. New York: Pergamon.

Hoch, E. L., Ross, A. O., and Winder, C. L. (eds) (1966). *Profesional Preparation of Clinical Psychologists*. Washington, D. C.: APA.

Kelly, E. L. (1961). Clinical psychology — 1960: Report of survey findings. *American Psychological Association, Division of Clinical Psychology Newsletter,* **14**, 1–11.

Kendall, P. C., and Hollon, S. F. (eds) (1979). *Cognitive-Behavioral Interventions: Theory, Research and Procedure*. New York: Academic Press.

Louttit, C. M. (1939). The nature of clinical psychology. *Psychological Bulletin*, **36**, 361–389.

Mahoney, M. J. (1974). *Cognition and Behavior Modification*. Cambridge, Mass: Ballinger.

Marmor, J. (1971). Dynamic psychotherapy and behavior therapy. Are they irreconcilable? *Archives of General Psychiatry,* **24**, 22–28.

Marmor, J., and Woods, S. M. (eds) (1980). *The Interface Between the Psychodynamic and Behavioral Therapies*. New York: Plenum.

Meichenbaum, D. (1977). *Cognitive-Behavior Modification: An Integrative Approach*. New York: Plenum Press.

Messer, S. A., and Winokur, M. (1980). Some limits to the integration of psychoanalytic and behavior therapy. *American Psychologist,* **35**, 818–827.

Palmer, J. O. (1980). *A Primer of Eclectic Psychotherapy*. Monterey, Calif.: Brooks/Cole.

Perry, N. W., Jr. (1979). Why clinical psychology does not need alternative training models. *American Psychologist,* **34**, 603–611.

Peterson, D. R. (1968). The Doctor of Psychology program at the University of Illinois. *American Psychologist,* **23**, 511–516.

Pottharst, K. E. (1970). To renew vitality and provide a challenge in training — The California School of Professional Training. *Professional Psychology,* **1**, 123–130.

Raimy, V. (ed.) (1950). *Training in Clinical Psychology*. New York: Prentice-Hall.

Rapaport, D., Gill, M., and Schafer, R. (1945). *Diagnostic Psychological Testing. Vol. 1*. Chicago: Year Book Publishers.

Swan, G. E. (1979). On the structure of eclecticism: Cluster analysis of eclectic behavior therapists. *Professional Psychology,* **10**, 732–739.
Wachtel, P. L. (1977). *Psychoanalysis and Behavior Therapy. Toward an Integration.* New York: Basic Books.
Wollersheim, J. P. (1974). Bewail the Vail, or Love is not enough. *American Psychologist,* **29**, 717–718. (Comment).

# Name Index

# *Subject Index*